Empath at the Office

**What Highly Sensitive People can do
to Manage Difficult Work-relationships,
Protect Their Emotions, and Create Inner Joy**

Aaron Kirchhoff

ISBN: 9781695410909

Editorial assistance: Beth Bazar
Cover design by Matt Davies
Interior typesetting by Vanessa Mendozzi

Special Thanks

I want to thank all my friends and family who have been so supportive of this idea. When I told them I wanted to write a book for sensitive people on how to deal with coworkers, the feedback was tremendously positive. So, thank you guys for the encouragement. It has helped motivate me to finish this project and share it with others.

Also, I want to thank all the difficult people I've worked with over the years. Your insensitive behavior forced me to grow and push myself to become the strong, joyful person I am today.

Contents

Preface

As this 15-year-old Swedish kid stood there yelling, threatening to sue me and the company for the red rash now covering his face, all I could think was, *This was not in the job description.*

I had been leading tours through national parks, Hollywood, Las Vegas, and other big tourist attractions for six months. This trip, however, was my first cross-country trek from Los Angeles to New York, with 15 Scandinavian teenagers from some private school abroad that I'm sure served lunch on gold plates. (The silver platter was reserved for afternoon tea.) Needless to say, there were copious bumps in the road, to put it mildly.

By day two of the three-week trip, some of the youths were already making it apparent that they intended to ignore everything I told them and instead look for ways to get beer. Once we reached New Orleans for swamp tours and beignets, however, one boy approached me with a red rash covering his face and neck. Before I had a chance to ask if he was OK, he shouted, rallied his classmates into a mob in the hotel lobby, and accused the establishment of having bedbugs. Hotel management, my boss, and several tour guides had to maintain order as these kids refused to stay there. I could hear a few individuals criticizing the tour as being "a waste of time," "terrible," and "the worst thing in America since potato chips on a sandwich."

I wanted to shout back, "I am doing my best, and I'm certain there are no bedbugs here! It looks like your rash is an allergic reaction. Also, what do you have against chips on a sandwich?"

The crowd of Swedish students eventually calmed down, and we proceeded with the tour. But I never heard the end of those bedbugs. The student with the rash was the most critical of the tour, of the food, and of my ability as tour leader. He made me feel self-conscious, and I questioned whether I was in fact doing a good job. Over the remaining two weeks, I fell into this gloomy cloud of self-loathing. It wasn't fun. *I'm not good enough. I'm a crappy tour guide. No one likes me. I should just quit. Why does this always happen to me?*

On the last day of the trip, after more than 1,000 miles of listening to my passenger complain about his itchy rash and the service on the trip, leaving me feeling personally responsible, he confronted me. His nonchalant gaze met mine as he boldly stated, matter-of-factly, "So it turns out my rash is an allergic reaction. I have a nut allergy, and I've been eating Nutella this whole time. Sorry."

Yeah, not in the job description.

Introduction

Let me introduce myself. My name is Aaron, and I'm just like you. I am a fan of the Marvel movies, I have a gluten thing but I still frequent Olive Garden for their breadsticks, and, like you, I'm an empath and highly sensitive person.

What Is an Empath and Highly Sensitive Person?

The terms I most identify with, if I had to choose, would be **empath** and **highly sensitive person (HSP)**. The lines seem to blur when defining these groups as both feel emotions deeply and share very similar characteristics, but, there are differences between the two. A highly sensitive person is hypersensitive to overstimulation. The noise, traffic, crowds and movement of people can be overwhelming for an HSP. Most empaths however, not only share this quality, but in addition, absorb the energy and emotions around them. Empaths sometimes have difficulty discerning between their own feelings, and those they take in from their environment. Most empaths are highly sensitive people, but not all highly sensitive people are empaths. (This book discusses many empath related issues, but will also provide helpful tips and techniques to be used by all people with varying degrees of sensitivity.)

The select group of people around the planet who share the descriptor of empath, have many things in common. We are creative and intuitive. Typically we feel recharged when alone and actively seek out time to ourselves, away from people. We thrive in solitude and feel depleted in large crowds. Empaths process information and emotions more deeply than most other folks and internalize all the stimulation we receive throughout the day. We have a natural gift for showing compassion and understanding for others and typically make great listeners.

An empath doesn't just show empathy for others; we absorb the energy and emotions around us like a sponge. If you're feeling sad, we become sad. When a friend is excited to tell us about the new Thai place down the street, we feel excited, too. We don't even have to talk to someone to feel their energy. When an empath walks into a room, they immediately *sense* what's going on.

Now, because empaths take in all the energy around

us, we have a tendency to feel overwhelmed and are more prone to stress and chronic fatigue. Think about it. As you're walking around all day, receiving constant input from TV, radio, commercials and ads, traffic, crowds at the store, people standing in the elevator, the smells of the dozen restaurants you pass on the walk to work, all the varying emotions of your coworkers, all their talking, e-mails, social media . . . you notice these things and more, and then try to process it all. It's complete sensory overload. By the time empaths drag our bodies back home, we are wiped out and drained—feeling heavy and bogged down, like a wet bag of sand. It takes all the energy we can muster to eat, get cleaned up, and put ourselves to bed, because the next day . . . it's back to work all over again. This is a problem for HSPs as well.

Because of the highly sensitive nature of empaths/HSPs, we also feel negative energy more deeply than most people do. We tend to take things personally, overthink things, and retreat into our own heads, replaying events over and over again. So when Tom at the office looks disappointed and we don't know why, we'll dwell on it all day, letting negative thoughts spiral without restraint.

Given what we now know about an empath/ HSP, isn't work, like . . . the worst place ever? All those people to deal with—and some of them can be mean. It's too much! Why can't some of us just stay home and earn a living as the Quiet Game World Champion?

Work Experience That Helped Shape Me into the Person Now Writing This Book

I have worked a lot of cruddy jobs and had to work with a lot of cruddy people. My work experience varies greatly, from fueling planes at the airport to working fast food, to teaching English as a second language, to being a microbiology technician—the list goes on for miles. The number of weirdos I've worked with stretches to the thousands, it seems, and as an HSP and empath, I've been steeped in all their energy. Every one of them. All of it, for years—like a faucet you can't turn off. I've been drowning in a bathtub of emotions for a long time.

One guy I worked with used to barge into me repeatedly with a leaf blower while we worked side by side, removing leaves from a yard in the fall. *Does he not see that I'm standing right here? Why does this keep happening? I deserve to have my own space!* I'd get so mad, my mood would ruin my whole day.

One time a manager at a fast-food restaurant told me how to use the fryer. I proceeded as directed. The next day she came face-to-face with me and screamed about how incompetent I was. After she threw some chicken tenders down in frustration, I wondered, *But I'm doing it just the way you showed me. Why am I here? What did I do to deserve such an outburst? Why are you so mean?* The shock of her shouting made me sink into a well of tension and anxiety so great that I started going to therapy. (I had already been planning to see a counselor. This was just another situation that further established the immediacy of my need for professional help.)

Late on a Friday afternoon in another job, my supervisor marched me into his office, sat me down with his boss on speakerphone, and abruptly informed me I could no longer work as a microbiology technician because I was falling behind. I felt like a boxer, dazed and swaying back and forth after a good punch to the gut. I felt, *I can't believe people here don't like me.* The supervisor politely opened the door and asked me never to come back. (In my defense, when I interviewed for that job, I thought it was to move boxes around or something, not to test food for *Listeria*. I got the job despite having no science background apart from watching *Stargate* in high school. So really, this is on them.)

After years of navigating the frigid wasteland of the workplace, struggling to fit in, to be happy, to be liked, to define how I was feeling and why I was so tired all the time, I finally wondered if I was missing something. Maybe the answer was with me? Instead of blaming idiots for being mean to me or cursing myself for being so sensitive, maybe there was a way to get stronger—to build my confidence and embolden my self-esteem. And boy, let me tell you, deciding to work on myself was like leaving the icy expanse of the Antarctic through a door to a sunlit beach paradise, complete with a swim-up ice cream bar and that Justin Timberlake song "Can't Stop the Feeling" playing on repeat! I felt like I was onto something important.

Deciding to work on myself was the best decision I ever made. I looked to the universe and said, "Hey, I get it. I'm a highly sensitive person and an empath, and I can feel every freaking detail around me, and it's too much. Instead of trying to run from it all, teach me how to face it. I can do this!"

I became much more self-aware. I started meditating every day to teach myself to be mindful of how I was feeling. I learned to watch my mind as an objective observer and realized our thoughts are a choice, not some horrid, uncontrollable avalanche destroying villages in its path. I was making progress.

I read every book. Watched every YouTube video.

Researched articles and listened to audiobooks. I filled a dozen spiral notebooks with ideas and thoughts on how to improve my life to become the best version of myself I could imagine. I had a lot of areas that I wanted to heal, but the area in which I've had the most success is dealing with people, especially at work. That's why I wrote this book.

I have completely changed my life around. If you were to look at me 10 years ago, you'd see a young man who never spoke up and who kept his head low to the ground. I was afraid and confused. I used to dwell on and absorb all the noise and negative energy at work. It used to control me and cause depression and anxiety. I thought there was something wrong with me, because people at work seemed to pick on me and treat me poorly. I struggled to find joy and meaning in it all, and I wondered if I'd ever be happy again.

But over time, I taught myself to be positive. I learned how to deal with people at work and manage all the noise. I found all these ways to ease my stress and calm down. I finally felt comfortable being a sensitive person and was actually excited for each day to begin. That's a big change from getting upset whenever someone sits too close on a bench. OK, I still don't like that! But it's like, *This whole bench is empty. Why do you have to sit right next to me?!* Anyhow . . .

I have learned a lot. So much, in fact, that I feel confident enough to share it all with you. I'm excited! Are you excited? I'm excited!

I know that I'm not the only empath out there who struggles with being around too many people. There are so many of us who share the same challenges, like how to deal with that obnoxious person at work, how to manage stress, and how to find happiness while going to a job you hate. All of these things I have dealt with, and still deal with in my life. But I am so much stronger now, and I want to teach others to be strong, too. Together, we can find ways to feel joy at work and manage the variety of people we see and energies we feel.

I'm so happy you picked up this book. It lets me know that I'm doing something right by sharing this information. It is my sincerest hope that you'll find something useful in the coming pages. My aim was to write a book that is a how-to manual for dealing with people at work. I wanted it to be easy to understand and filled with practical information that people can actually use. I hope you'll learn, accept, and apply many of these tools to help improve your perspective, not just at work and with your coworkers, but in life in general. Many of these tips, tricks, hints, and techniques, I use in other areas of my life, too. And I have seen massive improvement in my ability to cope with stress and manage my emotions.

I am not a psychologist or licensed professional in any way. I'm just a casual observer of human behavior who has the ability to sense emotion. After many years of accruing experience, research, and practice in becoming a better version of myself, I finally feel confident enough to speak up and declare, "I know what I'm talking about. And I want to help people."

This book is dedicated to the emotional, sensitive types of the world; the empaths, the highly sensitive people, the introverts; for anyone who has been labeled "too sensitive." To the people who have a hard time in crowds, who feel exhausted just from grocery shopping, and who have spent a lifetime fighting against subtle energy. If you feel overwhelmed by this world and all the noise in it, and you seek alone time to feel safe and let your guard down, this book is for you. If you want to improve your relationships with people, including your coworkers, this book is for you. If you're ready to grow, to release old, negative habits of thinking and become a stronger, more confident version of yourself, keep reading. I am so proud of you for taking the time and putting forth the effort toward increasing your awareness and building a better life for yourself.

So sit back, grab a cup of tea and a notebook and pen

(it can be useful to write down thoughts as you go), and tackle these chapters one at a time. You're a soldier for peace. A warrior. You're a sensitive person on the road to greater strength and well-being. Get after it!

1

Let Go of What You Can't Control

Ten years ago I was working in the oil fields of North Dakota, braving 100-hour work weeks in blizzards so thick I felt like one of those numbered balls in a lottery tumbler. I was 23 and working my tail off to save money for a volunteer trip to Africa.

My job was to maintain many pieces of large, noisy equipment, one of them being a horsepower unit. A huge tractor trailer carrying a big ol' engine on wheels was encased by pipes, hoses, and gauges all fitted together like this great metal octopus running on diesel. Fifty feet away from the horsepower units was the operation trailer, where several other crew members and I stayed inside, pushing buttons on glowing screens in the dark and kicking our boots against the floor to knock some feeling back into our frozen toes. One night, I was standing in this trailer with my crew when another coworker kicked the door in and slammed it behind him. I didn't have to be a psychologist to see he was in a bad mood. As he walked the length of trailer, he reached me, pushed me to the wall with his shoulder, and grumbled, "Get out of my way!"

I didn't deserve this. I was merely standing with my hands tucked in my pockets trying to keep warm when I was shoved to the wall offhandedly, as if I'd done something to cause offense. Regardless of having nothing to do with his bad mood, for days I was reluctant to talk to him because I thought he was mad at me.

Why does it seem that no matter where we work, there is always that one person? I'm talking about that person who is so angry at the world and at life in general that they feel entitled to treat you like garbage. Many people let this behavior roll off their shoulders and go about their day. But the sensitive people of world, the empaths, tend to let it bother us all day and even bring these thoughts home. The next day we see that same person, which brings back all the emotions and thoughts from the previous day, and the cycle continues. Soon those individuals don't even have to say anything; we just associate seeing them and being at work with those negative, hurtful emotions. It doesn't take long for the train to leave the station, your mind speeding toward negative thinking. Before you realize it, this person is triggering you at work all the time. And you didn't even talk to them today.

Getting to this point feels like being beaten down every day. Our sense of confidence goes downhill, and we begin lacking in self-worth. The mind wants to understand, *Why is this person so mean? What did I do to attract their hurtful comments? What is wrong with me?* The mind fights desperately, looking for a way to organize and "fix" the coworker's behavior.

This has got to stop! Don't dwell on what we can't control.

Empaths/HSPs tend to take things personally and internalize all the information in their surrounding environment. We prefer to think about things deeply, which is fine if all you're doing is deciding which T-shirt to wear to your friend's art show. But when it comes to analyzing mean and hurtful comments at work, we can lose ourselves in the details and slip into a hole of self-deprecating thoughts. *Stop that!*

I want you to recognize that your coworker's attitude and behavior are out of your control. There are so many reasons why some of the people we have to deal with are mean. Maybe they had a hard upbringing, and anger was the only way they could survive. Now, in adulthood, anger and hostility toward others is how they protect themselves from being hurt.

Perhaps your coworker is suffering from a personal matter and only knows how to express anger and stress by taking it out on others. By lashing out.

Maybe they're a bully and only know how to feel good about themselves by belittling those around them. They build themselves up by tearing others down.

Or maybe they got stuck in traffic, they recently got dumped, or the line was too long at Starbucks this morning and they didn't get their double-shot mocha latte, and they are just determined to let it ruin their whole day. (To which I want to say to them, "Brew your coffee at home and save the rest of us your temper tantrum!")

Whatever the reason for your coworker's attitude, the important thing to remember is, **it is not your fault**. If someone is a miserable person and all their words and energy are spent on negativity, take a cue from that Beatles song and "Let It Be." Simply acknowledge that this person is living in pain of their own, detach from it, and let it all go. You have better things to think about—like how amazing, beautiful, and talented you are! *Have you lost weight?*

So, if a coworker is a grumpy old fart who yells, gives

you the cold shoulder or silent treatment, corrects you constantly, or is standoffish, ask yourself, *What did I do to cause this behavior?* If they came to work like this and are taking it out on you, don't dwell on it all day. Let it be. Relax. Breathe and let it go. Breathe, relax, and move on.

Don't worry about what you can't control.
Drop it and let it go.

2

So You Work with a Blockhead

"I have a coworker who is just awful. She corrects me at every opportunity and says mean, hurtful things to me constantly. I've tried ignoring her, but that hasn't worked, and it's making it really difficult to do my job. What can I do?"

Scenario: The 12th floor of an office building in a bustling downtown cityscape. The entire floor is a sprawling honeycomb of shared desk space filled with the hum of printers and scanners, employees frantically typing e-mails, phones buzzing, and people walking to and fro. You, the sensitive, soft-spoken worker, are quietly reading e-mails and enjoying a midday banana when Larry, a nearby office-mate, leans over . . .

"You know you're not supposed to eat a banana like that. You're doing it wrong."

"What?"

"I watched a documentary about monkeys, and they peel it from the bottom, not the top. That's how you're supposed to do it. You're doing it wrong. Here, let me show you." Larry grabs the snack from your hand and peels from the bottom your already half-eaten banana and hands it back to you—as you think about how a moment ago you watched him pick his nose.

I didn't ask for your opinion, and now my banana is ruined. Thanks, Larry.

Ah yes, the old "I'm better than you, smarter than you, and more experienced than you, and you're gonna listen to my unsolicited advice. You're welcome!" routine. Have you ever worked with someone like this? It is so annoying! What is their deal?

I believe it has to do with their self-worth. People like this go out of their way to correct you or give unwanted help so they can feel better about themselves. They want to feel important, like they matter (which we all do), but they do it at the expense of others. If you're a sensitive person who works with someone like this, pay attention to their behavior and recognize it for what it is: their attempt to feel better about themselves. By finding ways to correct you, they are feeding their ego and giving themselves a temporary, inflated self-worth.

For empaths and HSPs, it feels like being stabbed in the chest with irritation. To us, it feels as if someone is pointing out all our shortcomings, all day, every day. How the heck can we be expected to come to work when there is always someone there to point out our mistakes? And a lot of the time, it's not even a mistake; they just want to prove that their way of doing things is better. *Your way isn't better; it's just different. Now, go sit down while I peel this orange.*

It hurts to have someone constantly tell you you're wrong. And this pain can make you doubt yourself, criticize other areas of your life, and spiral downward in a negative black hole that strips away your self-worth.

But it can get better. There are ways to improve how you feel at work. Through practice, you can block that coworker's negative energy and get to the point where you feel so good every day that their nonsense no longer bothers you. After learning some simple techniques, in fact, you may find yourself laughing more at work, because you see so clearly that this "evil" coworker has a weak sense of self, and you're much stronger than that. Woo-hoo!

Whether you're struggling with a coworker who is overly critical, mean, hurtful, or annoying, is just in a bad mood, suffers from Oscar the Grouch syndrome, or tries to peel your banana, the first step is detaching from their negative energy and letting it go. Like we talked about in the first chapter, it is not your job to carry around their awfulness on your shoulders. You can choose to elevate your thoughts and emotions through intention and focus.

Some techniques for dealing with difficult people:

1. **Increase your awareness through meditation.** Building a solid meditation practice every day will teach you to be more mindful of your thoughts and emotions. This is vital if you're going to pay attention to what your mind is doing, especially at work. Through this practice, you can catch your mind when it trails off in negative thinking spurred by something your coworker said. When you're at work, pay attention to what you're thinking. If you catch yourself thinking something negative or dwelling on something hurtful your coworker said or did . . . stop. Just stop and breathe. Say, "I see you, mind. I see that you're busy dwelling on these painful thoughts. I acknowledge these

thoughts and both love and accept myself." Simply recognizing and paying attention to your thoughts is, like, 80 percent of the battle right there! Congrats! By watching your thoughts, you bring them into the light, thus weakening their hold over you. This is a big step.

2. **Let it go.** (More on this in Chapter 7.) Take some deep breaths and detach from the negative, overwhelming energy around you. Recognize that your true, natural state of being is full of love, joy, and happiness. This natural state is much stronger than anything your coworkers can throw at you; you just have to practice living in this *good feeling* place. You can . . .

   - *Say affirmations.* Repeat: *I am strong. I am smart. I am good at what I do. I am confident in my abilities. I am powerful. I love who I am. I walk around all day like a prideful panther full of self-worth!* (Or whatever. The point is to feel empowered.) Use whatever affirmations resonate with you and get you feeling like the amazing, capable, wonderful person you are. Practice feeling so good that you take these emotions with you to work. Practice makes perfect. Keep your affirmations going at work. Write them on Post-its, set reminders on your phone, do things to remind yourself to stay in that *good feeling* place. You will see your coworker again, and she will continue to be who she is. You can't change that. You know this, so be prepared and be mindful of how you want to react. You can feel hurt and victimized, or you can focus on feeling confident, strong, and self-assured.

- **Visualize.** (More on this in Chapter 16.) Sit in a quiet, safe space at home and visualize being at work. Pretend you're going through the same eye-rolling conversation with this person who is being hurtful or correcting you for the thousandth time. What is she saying? How do you feel? Now, imagine you're in this new, natural state of being in which her comments don't bother you. How does it feel to have her criticism not faze you? Do you smile more? Do you laugh?

- **Try communicating and being honest.** (More on this in Chapter 15.) Roll out something like "Excuse me, but I don't need your help with this. If I have a question, I'll come to you." (If you've never spoken up before, your tormentor may be offended and taken aback. This is good! You're putting your foot down and practicing being assertive. Well done! She will likely stop a lot of her behavior because she will have learned that you don't put up with it anymore.)

There are many ways to handle the stress and negative energy you may absorb at work and from your coworkers, and we will discuss more of them throughout this book. In the beginning, just practice being mindful and separating your thoughts and emotions from the undesirable nonsense in your work environment. Choose to let those painful thoughts go and focus your mind on your preferred state of being—one of health, wellness, peace, and comfort. You can build strength, joy, and confidence from within that can grow and overpower all the hurtful energy you come across at work. All it takes is practice.

"What do I do about bullies?"

There are some people in this life who seem determined to be miserable. Whether they're mopping floors or managing a multimillion-dollar portfolio, they have made the decision to think and be negative. And what's worse, they seem to take that anger out on other people, and an empath/ HSP makes an easy target.

We all deal with anger and pain in different ways.

Through observation over the years, I've come to believe there are those whose coping mechanism for dealing with their issues is to put others down. I call this the bully mentality.

Think about those individuals back in grade school who seemed to pick on people constantly, the bullies. They said mean things, pushed the other kids around, and made fun of them. In some cases they were downright evil—like some kind of Nazi Darth Vader. Adolf Skywalker? I was not bullied incessantly in school, but I had my fair share of tough experiences. Some comments and hurtful behavior have left scars so deep, though, I am still dealing with them. So my question now is . . . why are some of my coworkers like this?

At an early age, the method some people learn in order to deal with their anger and low self-worth is to put others down. Doing so helps instill a false sense of superiority so they can feel better about themselves. **They build themselves up by tearing others down.** Bullies only know one way to feel better about themselves, and that is by ensuring that everyone around them is lower than they are. It's a terrible way to live—to hurt those around you so you can feel elevated for a short while.

One might take their negative comments and hurtful behavior and see it for what it really is: a cry for help.

These coworkers want to feel good. They're in pain and don't know a healthy way to feel good about themselves, so they lash out and hurt others. Once you begin to observe this, it helps to explain at least one possible reason for bully behavior in the workplace. With this realization, you may find it easier to start to feel more compassion toward bully coworkers.

I started to pity them—those jerks at work who so desperately want to prove me wrong, condescend, or criticize. This approach and new line of thinking helps me greatly in understanding mean people and has been a game changer in my life.

After looking at bullies and mean coworkers in this new light, try to show some empathy. This person who hurts you doesn't know any better—like a child. Without you there to push down, they can't lift themselves up. We all have issues we're dealing with, and some people don't know how to handle life in a healthy way. These bullies have to weigh down those around them so they can feel afloat in the rising waters of their insecurity, doubt, and lack of self-worth.

But you, the sensitive person, the empath, are a strong, independent thinker who knows how to boost your confidence and self-worth in healthy, productive ways, creating joy and love from within. Be patient with those who haven't caught up yet. Do your best to show compassion toward others.

Why do bullies seem to gravitate toward sensitive people? I think it's because our emotions are fragile and make for easier walls to tear down. Bullies don't want to work hard at feeling good; they are looking for instant gratification. Keep in mind, putting others down to build yourself up offers a very fleeting sense of elevated energy. They must keep at it to replenish the high they're looking for. Practice standing up for yourself (Chapter 15) so they learn not to mess with you.

3

I Am Worthy

Have you ever moved to a new place where maybe the kitchen counter sticks out too far at the corner? Every time you walk into the kitchen, your hip catches the sharp edge and you wince in pain. As the bruises start to accumulate, you curse yourself for hitting the same spot yet again. You look like you just joined the rugby team! But how many times does this happen before you remember to enter the kitchen differently? Only two or three, I'll bet. Now you sway your hips around the counter, narrowly missing it with the precision of a cat burglar navigating those red laser beams guarding glass-encased jewels.

When there is something in your life that is painful, often the first step to take is to ask, *OK, what can I change about myself to improve this situation?* You have picked up this book, so clearly you're doing just that. Bravo! This first step applies to all areas of your life, including dealing with people. Even though you can't control what people do, you can control yourself. How you think. How you feel. How you respond to this crazy world. You have the incredible ability to learn, to grow and improve yourself in so many different ways. So let's talk about growing and improving ourselves when it comes to dealing with difficult people.

If someone in your life is being mean or aggressive toward you—maybe a coworker drops snide comments, is critical of your work, or talks over you—make some changes in yourself. With this mentality of looking inward for answers, ask yourself, *What am I doing to create this behavior?* Remember, *"where your mind goes, energy flows."* If you think and feel negatively, the universe conspires to support that conviction by creating negative people and situations. It reflects back the energy you put out. This is called the Law of Attraction. So if you're experiencing people who treat you poorly, what thoughts or emotions do you have rolling around in your head that would be causing this? What energy are you putting out into the universe?

"Where your mind goes, energy flows."
—Ernest Holmes

If someone is treating you like you're not good enough, wonder, in what ways do you feel not good enough? Look at the people around you and describe to yourself how they make you feel. If their actions feel negative and hurtful, the next step is to look at your thoughts and really consider how these negative, hurtful emotions started in your mind.

Taking that first step to look inward and stop blaming others for your hurt feelings and instead take responsibility for your emotions is not easy. It is difficult to say, "I'm the problem. I need to change." It's much easier to look at someone, point, and say, "You did this. Now, fix it!" But if we're looking for a better life, to feel happy and create a new environment that is supportive and uplifting, the change has to begin from within.

So, with that in mind, one of the most common reasons people may treat you poorly comes from your own inner **lack of self-worth**. Look at your mind and be honest: What do you tell yourself every day? Do you say negative things? Is your inner voice a nonstop barrage of criticism and hurtful comments? Sensitive people have a tendency to keep a running monologue in our heads that is overly critical, self-deprecating, and full of pain. *I am not good enough. I am not strong enough. I can't do anything right. I am worthless. People treat me like trash.* The energy from these comments perpetuates itself and reverberates out into the universe. You are, in effect, attracting people and situations that help prove those thoughts to be true. The universe is always on your side. It wants to help you by giving you more of what you think about. Knowing this, it's time to change your thoughts to create a more agreeable reality.

Change your thoughts and your reality will follow.

Get in the habit of telling yourself awesome, amazing, beautiful, wondrous things that prove just how strong and special you are. Create a reality within you that evokes the changes you want to see from people.

Some affirmations to try:
- I am good enough.
- I am smart and capable.
- I deeply love and accept myself.
- I am amazing.
- I am worthy.

Next, come up with examples in your life right now that help prove these affirmations to be true. Make a list of ways that these positive thoughts feel real to you. Doing so will help reinforce the validity of this new internal monologue and start to make it a habit of thought.

> **Here's an example:** *OK, universe, I am worthy. I am good enough. I am strong. Well, how do I feel good enough? I can do so much! I can do things most other people can't, like ice skating. Yeah, that's a skill! Not many people are as good at ice skating as I am. Remember that first-place trophy I won when I was 10? I do! Who gets to do that?! I am awesome! And how many people can say they've been to Thailand? No one I know has been to Thailand, but I spent three weeks there volunteering in a school. That work was so fulfilling. And Alice said I was the best teacher they'd ever had! Look at all these things I can do. Oh, and just the other day, Jim complimented me on my e-mail and said it was well written. That felt really nice. I am good enough. I am worthy.*

The above example is a great way to show how the mind can find momentum from even the smallest things. Thinking about the ways you are good enough and worthy builds momentum. These feelings create more like them, and more thoughts come to you as positive emotion swirls and spins upward from within. You project this energy into the universe, and the universe says, "Oh, you're feeling confident and worthy today? OK, here are some people and situations today to help prove that's true." Keep your eyes open and watch little, positive things unfold throughout your day that reflect how you're already feeling inside. Life gets a little easier, step by step.

Today I made every green light on Spencer Avenue. Usually I hit every freaking one on red, and I complain about it, and by the time I get to work I'm in a bad mood. But today? Today I worked on myself and felt worthy and good enough in this world, and every light was green. Hmph . . . that was nice!

HOMEWORK

1. Come up with your own positive affirmations that make you feel strong, confident, and powerful and increase your self-worth. Be creative and see how different words and phrases resonate with you. Now say them to yourself—repeatedly.

2. Make a list of as many examples as you can think of that prove these positive affirmations to be true. For example, if you want to build up your self-worth, write down all the ways you feel worthy. What in your life makes you feel strong or like an expert? What are you good at? What are you proud of?

3. See if you can apply this method to your workplace. Come up with examples from work, no matter how small, that help prove you are worthy, smart, and strong. Focus on these instances and forget about the hurtful ones. Some examples:

   • I am the best at restocking and organizing the office supplies.

   • I delivered every package on my route so quickly, my boss was surprised I got back to the office early.

- I excel at customer service in my restaurant, and today that couple gave me an awesome tip.
- I installed that equipment all by myself. I feel proud about that.

Work on changing that inner monologue of yours to a more positive, supportive voice. Practice every day. Feel these emotions and take them with you to work. Look for examples throughout your day that help reinforce this new self-talk. Keep a journal at home that you update daily with "Here's what went right today," followed by a list of everything that happened as a response to your positive attitude. All of this is training your mind to focus on *good feeling* thoughts. By creating emotions that come from a strong sense of self, you send that out into the universe, which reflects it back to you. Life feels smoother. Things become a little easier in subtle ways. Then one day, those troublesome coworkers are no longer an issue.

Perhaps you get a new job. Or maybe your pain-in-the-neck coworker moves away, gets fired, or finally finds love through an online dating site and becomes a much happier human being. Whatever the case, it's the universe rewarding you for making the change you wanted to see. Now you can navigate your coworker's attitude, or a kitchen counter, with relative ease.

4

Quiet the Ego, Focus the Mind

"What do I do if I can't stand my job? It hurts so much going to work, I just want to quit and never go back." I was driving to work one day at a fast-food restaurant when I began having trouble breathing. My chest was so tight, and my vision was going dark—I was having a panic attack. I pulled over on the shoulder of the highway, rolled the windows down, and tried to catch my breath.

I went through a few more episodes like this at work that day, and I had to ask my boss if I could step outside. Standing there hiding behind a Dumpster, clutching my chest and holding back tears, I was confused, scared, and in pain. I wondered what the hell was happening to me.

I get it. Sometimes we get so low in life, it feels like we're suffocating under the pressure and strain of it all.

Even thinking about going to a job you hate can consume your senses and leave you weeping in your car, gripping the wheel tighter and tighter. This all-consuming pain feels like your heart is a dying star, pulling your body inward, collapsing your lungs, squeezing your muscles, and restricting your vision to the narrowest of keyholes. It hurts, this feeling.

Living an unfulfilled life tends to affect sensitive people more deeply, because their heightened senses make them acutely aware of their lack of joy.

If you're familiar with this suffering, I am here to tell you it's going to be OK. There is hope. Recognize what is going on here. You have become so focused on lack and pain that your mind is stuck in a repeating loop. Every day you repeat the thought habits of the day before. *I hate my job. I hate what I do. I'm in so much pain. Why can't I have _____? I hate my life.* This isn't you. This is the ego-mind running the show.

The ego is inherently displeased with everything and feels insecure. It wants attention and more things to make it happy. So, the nature of the ego is always to want something more. It is never satisfied, and it tricks you into thinking, *I need this and that to be happy. This job isn't good enough. I want. I need.* It wants things to distract it from its childlike insecurity, but each new thing offers only a temporary gratification before the ego says, *What about this over here? I want that! Gimme that!* And the cycle starts over.

The ego has a loud, obnoxious voice that is begging and screaming for your attention. But this is the important bit to keep in mind: You are a strong, willful being with power over your thoughts and feelings. The strength of your ego has only the power you give it, through your attention. Choose to let go. You carry within you a divine spirit full of infinite love, joy, and compassion—a well that never runs dry. No droughts or upstream dams here! The only difference lies in what you choose to think about. Do you enable your ego and give it attention? Or do you meditate, get calm, and be present, letting your reality just be what it is as you focus on love and laughter? Which one feels better?

So, in dealing with pain and suffering, if you feel completely overcome with hurt and sorrow about work and what you do for a living, just breathe. Let's change your perception to improve your mood and watch how life grows brighter. Strive to be unconditionally happy.

What is unconditional happiness? A state of being joyful and feeling happy, regardless of your environment.

How to Be Unconditionally Happy

This is the real trick to changing your life, improving your mood, and dealing with coworkers and other people. You will hear me talk about this throughout the book, because it is so incredibly important to the whole process and related to just about every tip and hint I have for you. This book is about dealing with coworkers, but these techniques can be used to improve all aspects of your life. When you become unconditionally happy, your life will start to change. Things you want will come to you easily, but it has to start with you.

So, to become unconditionally happy . . .

1. Build a meditation practice. Learning to meditate will help discipline your mind to let go and relax. It teaches you to detach from thoughts, to let them float past without engaging them. As your meditation practice grows, you train your mind to be aware of your thoughts. Bring this awareness with you everywhere you go, so you can catch your mind thinking about

unpleasant or negative things.

2. When you do catch yourself thinking unwanted, painful thoughts, drop 'em. Then and there.

3. Start thinking about things that bring you joy—things that make you happy and put a smile on your face. Focus your attention on fun, love, compassion, and laughter.

4. Feel the emotion attached to these new, positive thoughts and ideas. Describe these emotions to yourself in great detail. How do you feel? What brings you joy, and why?

5. Keep these good emotions with you at all times and practice thinking about them often. This is your good feeling place. With practice, you'll be able to call upon this good feeling place more easily. When you do, notice the magic happening. You are creating better-feeling emotions from within, not having to do with anything in your environment. You have just become unconditionally happy.

Your happiness is a choice you make every day. Through the power of intention, you can rise above your environment and feel happy—despite not liking your job.

This is a practice I do daily and am mindful of at every

moment. Building a strong meditation practice to improve your mindfulness is the first step. When you are conscious of what your mind is doing, of what you're thinking, you can drop destructive thoughts and actively steer your brain toward more joyful ones. At work specifically, notice when you're sad or unhappy, acknowledge your thoughts without judgment, and let them go. Then, actively remind yourself of how you'd prefer to feel. Bring back those feelings of joy and happiness and live in this feeling. Carry these joyful feelings with you during your day.

Now, you're no longer letting reality affect you. You're living from within and projecting positivity outward. Walking around the workplace in this Zen-like state is a game changer when it comes to finding happiness in life. You can feel happy even though you still have the same job. It all depends on what you choose to think about.

Oh, and remember, as an empath, emotion is your superpower. You have the ability to feel emotion more deeply than most. This also means you have a gift of creating powerful, *good feeling* emotions whenever you want! The path to being unconditionally happy is within you. All you have to do is feel it and live in that good feeling place.

But ultimately, if you honestly can't stand your job,

look for a new one. You deserve to be happy, and once you practice living an unconditional life, you can make better, more inspired decisions. If you feel it's time to move on from your current place of work . . . go for it! If changing jobs isn't an option right now because of commitments, bills, or whatever, get excited and start planning for a change as soon as possible. Life is meant to be enjoyed, and if you're spending the majority of your waking hours at a job that sucks the energy out of you, it is OK to reevaluate things. I know it can be scary changing jobs, especially if you've been there a while. The thought of changing jobs, working with all new people, and jumping into the unknown can be intimidating. Ask yourself where your priorities are. Would you rather stay at the same place that causes you pain, because it's familiar and the thought of leaving is too daunting? Or would you rather take inspired action to improve your life, braving the unknown and finding a better work environment?

Twenty years from now, don't you want to be able to say that you had the courage to stand up and fight for your happiness? Go for it! Upload your résumé on Indeed and get cracking!

5

How to Show Compassion

"But why should I show compassion toward someone who treats me so terribly? They suck so bad I can't stand them!"

I know, this is a hard one. Especially if they are downright mean and make your life so difficult. But showing compassion and understanding for your coworker is an important tool for letting go of the pain you've been holding on to and moving toward forgiveness. The act of forgiveness arises from a state of acceptance and love. Love for oneself and others. And keep in mind, love is a much more powerful state of being than hate, fear, or anger.

Show your coworker some empathy. As an HSP or empath, you're in the best position to show compassion and forgiveness, because emotion is your gift. Use it! You are the most capable of putting yourself in their shoes, feeling their pain, and observing how they suffer in their own way. Whoever they direct their stress and anger to, acknowledge that it comes from a place of suffering and do your best to be patient with them. They aren't on the spiritual self-improvement quest you are on and will take longer to reach their natural state of joy and being.

When I work with a bully, I always try my best to show compassion. Easier said than done when someone is screaming in my face. I can't always be that supportive, compassionate person I want to be in the moment. Sometimes I have to step back, take some time away, and remind myself to show them understanding. Someone who is irritating or pushes people around hasn't figured out a healthy way to feel good about themselves, and that leaves me wanting to send them more kindness, not bitterness.

I worked with a guy who talked constantly. He never stopped talking. We drove around town together mowing lawns and maintaining gardens. But he never stopped talking. The whole time we worked together, all I ever wanted was to drive in silence and be left alone. All he wanted was attention. I felt so much anger toward him. After a year of feeling like this, only when I'd given my two weeks' notice did I realize, "He's just looking for someone to care about him and his stories. No one ever talks to him." I finally felt more compassion for him and tried my best to become interested in his life. In his pet lizards. In what he cooked for dinner. In the jigsaw puzzles he put together . . . *Ohmuhgawd, do you ever shut up?* [Exhales, breathes deeply . . .] Compassion. Showing compassion.

Whether your coworker is mean, irritating, or hurtful to you in some way, try to look at things from their perspective. Get to know them better. It may help you understand them. Why do you think they act that way? Could it be they are in pain and trying to navigate this life, too?

Once, I tried to ask about a coworker's dog that he'd just adopted. "Mind your own business!" he barked. But this was OK. Instead of feeling hurt at his abrupt, admonishing remark, I felt warmth spread through my heart as I felt sorry for him. *Poor guy has no idea how to manage stress and anger.*

Showing compassion and patience for your coworkers is a strong technique in the workplace for letting go of your anger toward them. It helps put you on the path of forgiveness and focuses your mind on more positive emotions like empathy and kindness.

To show your coworkers compassion . . .

- Feel empowered by the fact that as an empath/ HSP, you're more capable of showing compassion toward others than most people are. In doing so, you move more quickly to feeling good yourself and letting go of your anger or hurt.
- Recognize we are all trying to navigate suffering to some extent, and we all have different ways of handling it. This lends itself to a feeling of "Hey, we're all in this thing together."
- Show them forgiveness. Say to yourself, *I forgive you. I recognize that someone would only say hurtful things if they themselves were living in pain. I choose to send you love and patience.*
- Reach out with an imaginary hand and comfort them on the back, shoulder, or arm. Imagine sending them love, even in times of anger and feelings of resentment. Showing love toward others instills a strong sense of love within you as well—giving and receiving. If you want to feel loved, first send love.

When attempting to show understanding for your coworker, the point of the exercise is to see where their own suffering comes from and identify with it as a commonality you both share—that we are all suffering to some degree. This is different from attempting to understand *what* they said or why you feel hurt. The latter feels more like dwelling on negative emotions, and we know that if we catch our mind doing this, we need to drop it and let it go. Overthinking a hurtful situation at work is just the ego's way of looking for justice because it feels victimized. Get back to that good feeling place and try again to show your coworker some compassion.

6

But I'm So Angry It Hurts

Anger is an emotion we're all familiar with. We have to put up with a lot of stress and weirdos in this life who cross us or make us mad. And with the variety of people in the workplace, I'm certain we have all felt angry at work for one reason or another. Have you ever felt anger toward a coworker so deep that it overwhelmed your thoughts for the rest of the day? You're not alone.

While working the closing shift at a Quizno's in high school, I heard a commotion in the stockroom in the back. I went to investigate, to find my coworkers arguing over this game. "I bet you can't do it!" one said. The other replied, "Oh yeah? I'll bet I can do it first try!"

"Hey, what are you guys doing?" I inquired.

They proceeded to explain that the game was to take a cup and fit it snugly in your pants, behind your belt buckle. Then, you would take a quarter, tilt your head back, and balance the coin on your nose. The trick was to try to drop the quarter into the cup without using your hands.

"Well, I can do that, give it here!" I beamed with confidence. I was 16 years old, and it was my first job. (Oh, to be young and naive again.)

I grabbed the cup and fit it into the top of my pants, tilted my head back, and placed the quarter on my nose. Just as I was ready for a test run, the front of my pants became drenched with freezing-cold water!

I recoiled in surprise and confusion, now standing there in soaked trousers. The uproar of laughter made it apparent that I wasn't in on the joke. I came to find out that the point of the game wasn't to drop a quarter into a cup, but instead to convince some poor kid to try it, and while his head was back, pour water down his pants. I should have taken note of the hole cut into the bottom of the cup.

My coworkers slapped me on the back and laughed so hard I thought they'd fall over. I didn't find it as amusing. As I got back to work and tried to get comfortable finishing my shift in wet clothes, I thought about how hurt, betrayed, and angry I felt. All I could think about was how angry I was that people do this to each other. *How could they do this to me? Why wasn't I smart enough to see it coming?* I was mad at them. At myself. At all people in general. I went to bed that night fuming like an active volcano.

Over the years I have become angry with coworkers for more reasons than I can remember. This stuff hurts, and I have always felt that I deserve better. I'm a nice person to everybody and expect to be treated the same way in return. And when that doesn't happen, I often get so mad I want to punch something!

This is not a good way to feel. Anger is such a low-feeling vibration, and dwelling on it only invites lower feelings, like hate, fear, and self-loathing. The more focus and energy you give anger, the stronger it becomes. So, the idea is to never let a negative thought or emotion overcome your natural state of peace and joy.

Recognize your anger, then let it go.

1. Have that good meditation practice in place to improve your mindfulness. When you are aware of your thoughts and emotions, you can manage them more easily and choose ones that better suit your well-being. Most people are completely unaware of what their minds are doing. They let them run from thought to thought like beagles chasing a scent trail. But with training, you can watch your mind and acknowledge to yourself,

Hey, I don't like this feeling. I see you, anger, and I acknowledge that you're here. I'm choosing instead to think about something that honors my well-being.

2. It's time to let that anger go. If you're at work and you recognize you feel angry, ask yourself, *Is thinking about this really worth my time?* Does it feel good to think about this anger? Pro Tip: It's not. Most things are so trivial, but our minds and egos make things bigger than they really are. When you decide it's not worth thinking about, just drop it. Remember, the idea is to feel good in life. You want to strive to get to a point where nothing in your environment can distract you from feeling good. Make feeling good a priority in your life. Being happy and joyful is your natural state of being.

One of the problems I see is that we tend to hold on to anger. We don't want to let it go. In many cases at work, when someone hurts you, you feel so angry you want to lash out. You want justice for what they did to you or how they treated you. I get it. It's a totally human way to feel. Mean people "deserve" to be punished, and until they are, you won't let go of your anger.

That's the ego-driven mind talking. It feeds on imbalance and craves drama. It is never satisfied and never gets enough attention. If you find yourself holding on to anger at work, recognize this as part of the ego. Notice the ego, your mind, trying to hold on for dear life, trying to get that revenge or justice it craves. Go back to being mindful, and recall the commitment you've made to feeling good in life and about yourself. Thinking about your anger and wanting justice will only create more anger and injustice within you. Whatever you think about grows, so let negative emotions go. I know it can be so hard to let go of the anger you feel when you want justice. But the healthiest thing to do is drop it and move on.

That commitment you've made to feeling good every day despite your surroundings is strong. It is much more powerful than hurtful comments or negative behavior at work. Do your best to remain focused on those *good feeling* thoughts that bring you happiness, and leave the rest behind. Anger will pop up again and again, but its voice will become less intense, dwindling down to a whisper. So remain focused and keep up the good work.

I used to dwell on anger all day, bring it home, take it with me to bed, and then pack it up to take back to work the next day. I was miserable. After some practice and mindfulness, however, I changed my life. The following example is what my mind does now.

Example: Something happens at work that makes you angry.

God, I'm so angry at this person. Why is he like this? He is so mean and hurtful, I hate coming to work. I wish this person would just get fired already! Hey, wait, I've been thinking these angry thoughts for over an hour. Whoa, my mind took this and ran with it, didn't it? Hmm. I am better than this. Didn't I decide to be unconditionally happy? Oh yeah, I did. I know that thinking about this halfwit at work, even for a second, sends me spiraling, so why do I even bother? It is not worth thinking about if it's not constructive and doesn't help me feel good about myself. That's right, I remember now. I can't see a way I can benefit from thinking about how angry I am, so I'm done.

Lord/universe/infinite God/wisdom, I'm dropping this entirely and getting back to good *feeling thoughts. Let me think of three things right now that bring me joy. Ummm . . . I can't wait to get off work and watch the next episode of* Umbrella Academy. *I am so thankful for my new car. I've wanted it for so long; this is awesome! And I'm so glad I packed a delicious and healthy lunch today. I'm going to feel so great after I eat it. Oh, and I love that I had a good conversation with my friend last night. We laughed so much. Hey, that's four things I'm thankful for! I love that when I focus on happy, positive things, my mind spirals upward. So cool! OK, time to get back to work. I feel better now.*

And that's my mind at work now.

If you feel anger toward someone at work, catch yourself feeling this way and actively try to let it go. It does you no good to wonder, scheme, or overanalyze what they did or what was said, even if you feel in the right. Thinking about it will only create more of the same negative emotion. Now that you know energy flow begins in your mind, isn't it much nicer to choose better-feeling thoughts?

"But I want them to pay for what they did."

I know it hurts. You want to hold on to thinking about this pain until somehow your coworker is punished and good triumphs over evil. It feels as if your top priority is seeking justice. But holding on to that anger only really hurts one person: you. Be kind to yourself and let it go. I believe the universe is watching, and those poor souls who cause trouble at work and make everyone miserable will continue to create more pain for themselves until they wake up and grow in a spiritual way. Until then, don't share in their misery. Stop holding on to your anger and let it be. Make feeling good the top priority in your life, so much so that no anger is ever worth holding on to.

7

How to Let Go

It is so important to learn how to let things go. If you're anything like me, you can dwell on something negative until it makes you sick. Developing the skills to acknowledge things in your life that you want to let go of and then release them takes time and practice, but you can do it! Be patient with yourself, though. You can't watch that *Free Solo* documentary and expect to climb Mount Everest tomorrow. It takes time. Growing and improving yourself is hard work, so remember to be kind to yourself.

The first step is to be mindful of your thoughts and emotions. Pay attention to when something is upsetting you and acknowledge it. Shining a light on your problems releases a lot of their energy and power over you. Just by seeing the negative energy we're focused on, we detach from it and halt the runaway train of thoughts in the mind. This is half the battle right there, just watching your thoughts. Instead of letting your mind bounce from topic to topic and analyze things from your ego's point of view—from a standpoint of lack, insecurity, and victimization—you can stop all that by simply acknowledging that it is happening.

It really is like shining a spotlight on a burglar who's been hiding in the shadows. He only has power if he can't be seen, so this sudden attention scares him off. The ego is the same way. It wants to creep around undetected, trying to run the show. But you've made the commitment to be aware. To be mindful. You're working toward a new, happier, more balanced you. And it all starts with watching the mind.

Once you've noticed that something negative is bothering you and how it makes you feel, it's time to let it go. Accept what it is you'd like to release, then imagine it slowly disappearing from existence.

Here is how to practice letting things go:

1. **Meditate.** Sit in a quiet, peaceful place and just practice following your breath in and out. Clear your mind and let go of any thoughts. Simply focus on your breath. Clearing your mind feels good, and you'll notice that you start to think less and less. When thoughts or ideas

come up, catch your mind trying to wander in that direction and gently pull your attention back to your breathing. Feel this calm, meditative state deeply and give thanks for being able to feel at peace.

2. **Visualize.** While meditating, it's often helpful to visualize the pain and anger you're holding on to. Using your imagination, try to picture what this painful emotion looks like inside you. Does it have a shape? Does it have a color? Use some adjectives to describe it to yourself in detail and explore how it makes you feel. Then, imagine that this negative thought or emotion is coalescing in front of you. Feel it leave your body and build into some form or object outside of yourself. You're still meditating, breathing, and feeling calm. With every exhalation, you feel a little more of this pain leave your body and watch it join this free-floating mass in front of you. There are no wrong answers as to what you see. This is your imagination. Do you see a black, flowing mass of negativity? Is it floating or sitting on the ground? How big is it? Does it have a distinct shape, or does it seem to flow and change? Watch this energy but don't cling to it. It is outside your body now, and you can observe it without getting attached. Mentally wave at it and say, *Hiya, buddy!*

Now, picture opening your arms and giving yourself permission to let this go. Imagine the object in front of you that represents your pain, anger, fear, and worry, and surrender it to the power of the universe. Watch as it dissipates or floats away, until you can no longer see it anymore. It is completely gone. Now, how do you feel? (This is one of my favorite techniques for letting things go.)

You can even ask for help. As you're imagining letting go of this pain, pray to the universe/God/the energy force/your higher self (whichever you feel most comfortable with) for help. Say, "Here it is. Here is this hurt I've been holding on to. It no longer serves my highest good, and I'm choosing now to let it go. I surrender this pain and have faith that you will help me. Thank you for your guidance." Then imagine it just wafting away into nothingness.

3. **Say affirmations.** Make a list of sayings and phrases that help you emphasize how you want to feel when confronted with pain or negativity in the workplace. These will be different for everyone, and you can alter the wording until you land on something that works for you. The point is to pay attention to how these phrases make you feel. Choose the affirmations that resonate

with you the most and repeat them as often as you like. Some examples are . . .

- This no longer bothers me.
- I am strong.
- I feel above this today.
- I choose to let this go.
- I release this.
- I feel good in this moment.
- I deeply love myself.
- I am confident.

4. **Get back to that good feeling place.** Now that you have actively let this negative energy go, it's time to replace those thoughts with something more constructive, right? Think about that good feeling place you love so much. Be reminded of how you'd prefer to feel again and live in that state of happiness and comfort. Create an infinite pool of love and compassion within you that feels more powerful than any hurtful comment at work. Make your priority at work to feel good, no matter what. Decide that nothing, no matter how hurtful, can derail you from feeling good.

5. **Learn the emotional freedom technique (EFT).** EFT is a relatively new concept that is making its way into Western understanding and practice. The idea is that

energy is all around us. It makes up everything and everyone, and therefore we are energy, too. Our bodies, full of this life force/energy/aura, have meridians or hot spots that can be influenced and acted upon by tapping certain parts of the body. By gently tapping these energy points on the body (such as the wrists, temples, and top of the head), one can stimulate the flow of energy, release blocks, promote healing, and help with mental and emotional growth, like aiding in releasing negative thoughts and emotions. I have tried EFT and love it! If you'd like to learn more, I recommend a number of authors on the subject, including Nick Ortner and Dawson Church.

Letting things go is hard work. Often, things will pop up that threaten to throw you off your game. Don't get discouraged. Congratulate yourself for being one of the few who are trying to do better. You're amazing! If you do have a bad day and can't seem to let something go, it's OK. This is totally normal, and we're all going through the same thing—trying to be better. I doubt any masters or gurus out there have reached a point where nothing bothers them. Even the guru on the mountaintop must have to fan away a mosquito now and then. It's a lifelong practice. But it does get much easier with time. Use these techniques, learn new ones, and become the best version of yourself that you can—one who rises above all the negativity at work and elsewhere.

8

What If I Can't Let It Go?

This is why it's called a **practice** instead of a finish line, where we're perfect at all things. Our minds don't want to stop thinking, as if we were addicted to it. It's no wonder letting something go is so difficult.

As I write this chapter, I'm sitting in a coffee shop. While waiting in line to get my hot cup of decaf, I noticed that the person behind me was standing just too close to me. It felt like an invasion of privacy, and I wanted to say, "Hey, you, can't you see my invisible bubble of personal space? Back off!" I thought about saying something, but I'm passive-aggressive by nature and don't like confrontation. I said nothing and inched forward, only to have them move closer. Then my mind gained speed, barreling downhill in negative thoughts. *Why does this bother me so much? Why am I so sensitive? Do other people go through this? How can this person not feel how uncomfortable it is to stand this close to someone?* Now I'm trying to calm down and write about what to do when you can't stop thinking about things . . . as I'm going through it myself.

An HSP loves to analyze and think things through. That's good when you're lost in the woods and you need to know which direction to go. But when a coworker says something to upset you, it's important not to get hung up on negative thinking. That's why we practice letting it go and focusing on the positive nature of our true, inner selves. However, we can't just snap our fingers and be magically whisked away to the land of Oz. It takes work— hard work—to be able to let things go. And some days are just harder than others. Sometimes, in the moment, we can't let it go. We're in too much pain. The mind will dwell on these thoughts, jumping from one to another like an uncontrollable lightning bolt in a summer storm. Next thing you know, you're having a terrible day, and everything is just the worst. If this sounds familiar, you're not alone.

If you're at work and something sets you off, maybe a coworker criticizes you in some way, or your boss is a jerk, or someone just stands too close to you at Panera, many times we can't help but think about it. And think about it. And think more about it. And this thought that started like a cough in a quiet library is spreading now like an infection. You see your mind trying harder, going deeper into this mess of negative thinking. You're fighting for that good feeling place, but it's just not happening. This brings up more anger and guilt, and thus the ball keeps tumbling down the rabbit hole.

First of all . . . breathe. Just breathe. It's natural to feel hurt or annoyed by these things, and our feelings are totally valid. You're not going crazy. Your mind has just latched on to negative feelings and emotions today and won't let go. If you've recognized this, good for you! Remember, being mindful of your thoughts is the biggest step. You may not like what your mind is doing at this moment, but at least you're aware of it.

Next, if you've tried letting it go, if you've done the work to relax and breathe and focus your mind on that good feeling place but it's just not working, let's try something different.

Get distracted. Distract your mind with something so you're not dwelling on painful thoughts. Get busy doing something so you're not thinking so much.

Damage Control

Step 1: Recognize what you're thinking about and how you feel. If it's irritating or hurtful, try to let it go.

Step 2: If letting it go isn't working, drop it by doing something else.

- Watch a movie or TV show.
- Sleep.
- Cook something.
- Clean the house.
- Call a friend.
- Do art: paint, draw.
- Go to the gym.
- Do a puzzle.
- Listen to music.
- Play a game.
- Sew something.

What are your hobbies? What do you love to do? Make a list of things you like to do that keep your brain busy with something. I enjoy playing solitaire sometimes. It's easy, quiet, and something completely mindless that I can do on my own. It keeps my hands busy and my mind focused on the game. This simple trick lures my mind away from dwelling on terrible coworkers or other negative thoughts, and I start to feel better. After an hour, if I still feel down and my mind is still reeling, I segue to other distractions. I focus on having fun and enjoying my time. I do anything I can to feel better and keep my mind off work or whatever is bothering me. Eventually, I calm down and can meditate and clear my mind so I'm back in that good feeling place again.

I'm careful not to judge myself too harshly, either. Some days I can find peace quickly. Other times it can take a full day or more to distract my mind before I'm ready to try again to feel my preferred emotions. If it's a week, then a week it is. No judgments. I show myself only patience and compassion. I don't judge myself if I can't feel calm or joyful like I've been practicing. Instead I say, *Hey, I see that I'm not happy right now, and that's OK. I forgive myself. Let me find something else to do, and I'll come back to my mindfulness practice when I'm feeling better.* Then, whatever it is that's really bugging me, I just drop it. Totally and completely. Because I know thinking about it is only making it worse. So I let it be.

Two important notes:

1. **Don't try so hard.** Yes, letting go of negative emotions is important, but not if it feels like you're fighting with yourself. The aim here is to feel relaxed, relieved, at ease, and peaceful. If you're battling to let something go, and it feels like a struggle, don't force it. Be calm. Take a deep breath and drop it. Get busy doing

something you enjoy and take your mind off things.

2. **Forgive yourself.** Remember to take it easy on yourself. Watching your mind and focusing your thoughts takes time and practice, and it is not easy. It's not like we can flip a switch and say, "OK! I'm better now!" That'd be nice, huh? No, we are all trying the same thing here, and we are all going to have days when we can't let things go. It's OK. Show yourself kindness and patience, and come back to the practice of letting go when you're feeling better. No rush. Only love.

In summary, if you can't stop thinking or can't let something go, drop it by distracting yourself with an enjoyable activity. Come back to your mindfulness practice when you feel better.

> "No problem can be solved from the same level of consciousness that created it."
>
> Albert Einstein

9

Congratulations, You're Sensitive!

On my good days, being an empath/ HSP makes me feel empowered, uplifted, and excited to be alive. I am aware of all my senses and give thanks for my favorite things in life. But on my bad days, I curse the heavens for my increased sensitivity. Feeling so drained and overwhelmed all the time leaves me in what seems like a chronic state of defeat. I scold the universe and ask, "Why am I like this? Being sensitive makes life a million times harder!" On these days, it's important to remind myself that although there are extra challenges for an empath, being sensitive is a gift.

If you're a sensitive person and are feeling like life is too much to handle, when the stress of the day is piled on the stress from the day before and everything starts to become overwhelming . . . take a beat. Breathe and relax. Think about how less than one percent of the population have the extrasensory perception to absorb and feel emotion. It can be a strain sometimes, but you can do things most people can't. Take a minute and consider it a gift. Be grateful. This will help to strengthen your self-worth and confidence and help turn your mood around. Here are some ways that being a highly sensitive person or empath is a gift.

1. Sensitive people make great listeners. No one can listen and understand like an empathic, sensitive person.

2. People love being around confident, sensitive people. You have good, attractive energy, and subconsciously people are drawn to you. By nature you help improve people's energy, simply with your presence.

3. Navigating this world using emotion is like having a sixth sense. You can make better decisions at work, in your personal life, with relationships . . . All areas of your life can improve when you trust how you feel and follow your gut.

4. Very closely associated with *feeling* is *knowing*. The empath has strong intuition and knows things before other people do. When you need answers, you can call on this higher knowing to guide you. A great

book to get you started on improving your intuitive ability is *The Intuitive Way*, by Penney Peirce.

5. You're perceptive and pick up on things most people are too busy to notice: the texture of an old oak desk, the subtle vibration in the ground preceding your morning train commute, the smell of a coffee shop on a brisk morning. This attention to detail aids in paving the way to staying present and getting to that good feeling place. You're naturally gifted in meditation, too.

6. You feel emotions more strongly than others do, which means you have a greater capacity than most to feel the good ones: joy, fun, excitement, love, passion, intimacy, amusement, fulfillment, creativity . . .

7. You're more sensitive to discomfort and unhealthy, out-of-balance situations, which means you notice them more quickly than other people do—and that is the first step toward changing those situations.

8. Being sensitive gives you the ability to be a great communicator, because you're in touch with how you feel inside. You are better able to articulate emotion, and therefore you can relay honesty and clear, concise information that people can understand.

9. Highly sensitive people and empaths tend to be

amiable and to get along with others.

10. Sensitive people are the creative types—the painters, musicians, actors, poets, writers, photographers, and artists showing this world how to feel. Without you, there'd be far fewer street performers on Venice Beach. And a lot less heart, too.

HOMEWORK

What other ways can you think of in which being sensitive is a gift? Write them down and display them on a wall at home to remind yourself every day how gifted you are.

10

How to Manage Stress

Stress at work can be a strain on the mind and the body. It can mess with your emotions, and HSPs and empaths feel emotional highs and lows like a yo-yo as we struggle to understand what the heck is happening. Stress is weird like that. It can make you feel depleted, angry, exhausted, manic, overwhelmed, teary eyed, or anxious. It can manifest itself in your body physically as headaches and sore or stiff muscles. Without a healthy way to release this tension, it can lead to even worse physical ailments like illness or disease. Have you ever worried yourself sick? That's stress presenting itself as a physical symptom that started as thoughts in your mind.

Stress can make empaths/ HSPs feel like we're losing our minds as we try to cope with the constant barrage of noise, people, movement, and the demands of the workplace. What's more, feeling this way has become a normal state of being for many, because they think, *Well, this is work. It's supposed to be stressful. I just have to suffer.*

It is common for many to spend years, maybe their whole lives, dealing with adverse working conditions, subjected to very demanding circumstances, with no idea how to feel better. We all want to feel better at work, but most people either don't even realize they've been living life in stress mode, because it has gone on for so long, or they do know they're overwhelmed at work but have no clue what to do about it.

In addition, for many empaths and HSPs, being around people all day is utterly exhausting. We thrive in solitude and feel depleted in crowds and even small groups, so working with others for an extended period of time is very hard. By the end of the day, we feel drained—as if our battery has turned over but the engine isn't running. It can seem like every day at work is hard, and you know it's going to be hard, so you don't want to go. So, on top of the regular stress of the workplace, an empath/ HSP must handle the onslaught of stimuli coming in from all sides—all the energy and emotion around them.

It's no wonder sensitive people feel constantly wiped out and exhausted and have a really tough time dealing with stress.

"I can't stand my job! It hurts too much. The people
are mean. I hate what I do. I'm so tired of feeling tired
and overwhelmed, I can't take it!"

But this can change. You don't have to quit your job just
yet to see improvements in your attitude and energy levels.
This rut of daily torture can change. But it has to start with
you. Begin with some coping strategies for getting through
the day. Do your best to follow your greatest and highest
self and feel as good as possible.

**Stress Management Ideas for Work and Home (Practicing
Self-Care)**

- **Do deep-breathing exercises.** If you're feeling
  stressed at work, try a deep-breathing exercise. Sit
  down, relax your shoulders, relax your neck, feel the
  weight of your body sink into your chair, and get comfortable. Slow your breathing and inhale to a count of
  6: *in, 2, 3, 4, 5, 6* . . . Then exhale: *out, 2, 3, 4, 5, 6* . . .
  And again. Inhale: *in, 2, 3, 4, 5, 6* . . . And exhale: *out,
  2, 3, 4, 5, 6*. Take long, deliberate breaths. Do this 10
  times and see how you feel. Watch your body relax

even more deeply and feel your mind clearing. Every time you exhale, imagine you're breathing out all the stress, tension, and panic you may be carrying. With each inhalation, imagine taking in beautiful, golden, healing energy that makes you feel replenished like taking a sip from a mountain stream. Practice this breathing technique at home, at work, and in your car, and it will come to you more easily the next time you call upon this trick—just like riding a bike.

- **Take a nap.** Sleep is just great!
- **Listen to calming nature sounds.** Find some time to put on headphones or earbuds and listen to recorded nature sounds. There are plenty of apps for your phone and a plethora of YouTube channels dedicated to calming, meditative sounds and music. Many empaths/ HSPs are sensitive to noise, so not only does this technique help bring you into a relaxed state of being, but it also helps drown out the loud, bustling nature of the work environment so you can focus. Some of my favorite nature sounds I listen to through the app on my phone include gentle rain on leaves, a crackling campfire with crickets and frogs, and a flowing stream with bird songs.
- **Take breaks for alone time**. An empath/ HSP tends

to feel overwhelmed around a lot of people, so quiet alone time is a great way to recharge and get energized again. Depending on where you work, it may be tough to find time alone. So, set aside time just before work, or right after, to sit, get still, and clear your mind. You can try sitting in your car. Walk around the building alone. Go to the bathroom if you have to for a few quiet moments. Find a supply closet or a quiet corner where you can rest and be yourself. Be proud of yourself for taking time out of the day to practice self-care. Be grateful for this moment of solitude and look forward to the next one. Not every job allows time to yourself. This sucks. With a little bit of mindfulness practice, however, you can carry the feeling of being alone with you, even though you may be surrounded by people. Find time alone when you can, pay attention to how you feel in those moments of solitude, and live in those emotions at work.

- **Go for a walk.** Walking is such a simple exercise but a powerful one. Your body was built to move. Get into action! Put one foot in front of the other for 20 minutes a day and it can have a profound effect on reducing stress. It relaxes and loosens muscles, helps clear your mind, and gets energy flowing throughout your body. When you become stressed at work, plan a short walk; even 5 minutes is better than nothing. Whether it's on your lunch break or later in the day, walking will help.

- **Do grounding exercises.** See Chapter 12.
- **Practice yoga, stretching, or tai chi.** Set aside time first thing in the morning to stretch for 10 minutes. It makes a world of difference for reducing stress, as it helps loosen stiff muscles but also improves overall mood. You can even take a yoga class or learn tai chi to help calm your body and mind and sink into deep relaxation.
- **Take your mind off things (distract yourself).** See Chapter 8.
- **Go to your car and yell.** Here's a nice cathartic technique for you to try. Stress builds up inside us like a party balloon, and it can pop if we don't find ways to release this pressure. We can become irritable and angry and feel mean living in a state of overwhelming stress. So it is important to our overall well-being to invent ways to find relief from this pent-up stress. Screaming in anger at your coworkers is not recommended, but if you can find a place where you won't get weird looks . . . go scream your head off! Yell as

loud as you can! The act of yelling and shouting feels like a great release of tension and angry energy. When you express yourself in this way, it's like opening the release valve on a gas line—it can be very constructive when you're experiencing great amounts of stress.

- **Sing it out.** Similar to the previous management tool of yelling, singing is another way of using your voice to express yourself that helps relieve stress. If you're afraid to sing in front of other people, sing in the shower. Sing in your car, on your daily walk, or in your bedroom. Look for opportunities to belt out your favorite tune and sing it loud and proud. See if you can feel any stress leave your body as you sing. If this helps, keep it up! Put on your favorite Disney soundtrack and crank it to 11!

- **Listen to music.** Just listening to music is an awesome way to relieve stress. Music has a tremendous ability to stir emotion and affect our mood. Choose some upbeat tunes or whatever music you love that makes you feel better and more calm and at ease. If it's allowed, listen to music during the workday.

- **Listen to audiotapes or podcasts**. Download a guided meditation that you can listen to at work. Or listen to podcasts that talk or audiobooks that make you feel calm and relaxed. They can be self-help books to teach you something, or just good stories you enjoy listening to. Whatever you choose to plug into, let it send you into a calm, relaxed state.

- **Exercise.** Just as walking helps relieve stress by getting your body moving, any physical activity helps reduce stress as well. Buy a gym membership and get that blood pumping! Many people associate going to the gym with trying to lose weight. Try instead to focus on just feeling good. The aim here isn't to achieve that perfect body image; worrying about that only creates more stress. Exercise with the intent to feel good, to feel the energy flowing through your body and boost your mood. You'll feel the weight of stress fall off your shoulders, and perhaps without worrying about losing weight, you may find that that starts to fall off, too—*if that's a goal of yours.*

- **Get a massage.** Another great way to relieve stress is a massage. Your muscles carry a lot of tension from various stressors in the day-to-day, so relaxing them helps release that tense energy. Have your partner give you a back rub when you get home. Or just sit on the living room floor and spend some time rubbing and massaging your own legs, feet, arms, shoulders, neck, and scalp. Spend the time necessary to relax your body and ease your mind. Make an appointment to visit a massage therapist and see if a professional can help you. There are a number of different massage techniques out there to try, so take care of your muscles; ease the tension within them and your mind and spirit will follow.

- **Cry.** Crying has a societal stigma attached to it, as if crying were a sign of weakness. Nothing could be further from the truth. Crying means you're in touch with how you feel. You're connected with your emotions and are expressing the inner you. Whereas other people feel they need to stifle their true nature, you are connected with your inner self. You are living closer to all those good feeling emotions like love, joy, and compassion. So crying, I feel, is a good thing. A necessary thing. If you feel the need to cry, go for it. Find a quiet, comfortable place like a restroom stall or somewhere else out of sight where you can let your guard down. Crying is healthy and serves as a form of self-expression that aids in reducing stress at the workplace. And when you cry, take comfort in the fact that it requires great strength and courage to show that amount of vulnerability. Not everyone is strong enough to cry.

- **Write about it.** Again, finding ways to relieve stress so you're not holding on to it is the key here. Writing down your thoughts and feelings is a great form of self-expression to help reduce stress. Start a document on your computer or buy a journal and some pencils and get cracking. There are no wrong ways to start writing down how you feel. You'll be amazed how quickly the ideas flow once you open up to expressing yourself through writing. No one is ever going to read it, so feel free to write without restraint.

- **Talk about it.** If you're feeling an insurmountable level of stress, don't keep it to yourself. Find someone to talk to. Confide in a close friend or family member. Tell them how you feel and what you're going through. Hopefully this person is a good listener and will offer constructive support and love. You want someone who makes you feel comfortable and with whom, when you're finished talking, you feel much better—like you got a laundry load of emotions off your chest.

You may find that professional counseling is the way to go. That's great! A licensed professional can offer constructive hints and tips to help you get through the tough times. Finding someone to talk to reduces stress, because as you talk, you're releasing all those pent-up emotions and frustrations and getting them all out of your body.

- **Meditate.** This is one of the best decisions you can make for your overall well-being. Meditation helps relax the mind, calm the spirit, and put the body into a state of relaxation. If you've never meditated before, give it a try. Download one of the many apps (I use Calm.com) to your phone and learn with a basic, guided meditation. Meditating teaches you to quiet your mind so you can watch your thoughts and be mindful of what that brain of yours is doing. In monitoring your mind, you can detach from negative thinking, reduce stress, and choose thoughts that are conducive to better feelings.

- **Say affirmations.** Having a half-dozen-or-so affirmations you use to cope with stress helps put your mind back into that good feeling place of joy and peace you keep practicing at home. When you're at work and feel very stressed, try saying to yourself, I am calm. I am completely at ease. I love being here and now. I deeply love and accept myself. I am so full of love. *I am completely relaxed. My shoulders are heavy and calm. My breathing is sloooowwwwww and steady*, and so on. Have these affirmations written down on a piece of paper, on Post-it notes, in your phone, wherever is the easiest to access them to quickly remind yourself, *Hey, I don't want to feel stressed out. I would rather feel like this!*

- **Make a gratitude list.** Here's a really powerful technique to help guide your frame of mind away from stress and back toward positivity. Sit down with a pen and paper and list the things you're truly thankful for. How many ideas can you think of? What are the things you're most grateful for? Sometimes, when we're really stressed and feeling low, it can be hard to find things to appreciate in life. But these moments of difficulty are exactly why you want to change in the first place. Use this as motivation, start slow, and just name a few things you're grateful for. They can be small things, like how much you enjoyed that coffee and doughnut this morning, or how nice it is to just sit back, watch TV, and do nothing. Start naming little things you're grateful for and watch as your mind starts to grab at every little thing, every spark of happiness you have in your life, no matter how small.

Once the ball gets rolling, you may find it hard to

stop. This is good! There is so much to be thankful for. We spend so much time feeling stressed and tired and wanting things to change that we forget to appreciate what we have. Take some time to create a list of things you love about your life. Keep that list with you and look at it often. Add to it. Then really, and I mean really, think about how those things make you feel. Joyful? Appreciative? Relieved? Positive? Carry those emotions with you like a trophy above your head, higher than all the stress and nonsense of the workplace.

- **Look at pictures that make you feel happy.** Pretty straightforward, right? When you're feeling stressed out or angry, take some time to look at pictures that make you feel good. What do you love to do? What are your hobbies or interests? If you have a phone or computer nearby, take some time to scroll through photos that make you feel more at ease. These images should help stir your imagination into the good feeling place and reduce stress in the process. Some examples could be pictures of your loved ones, sunsets, puppies or other baby animals, gardens, the ocean, William Shatner, a calm forest, or a rainy day. Maybe make a vision board showing all the things you love in this world, then take a photo of it and keep it with you. Be creative.

- **Use a Himalayan salt lamp.** Pink Himalayan salt is said to have healing properties like absorbing negative energy and promoting a calm, peaceful atmosphere. These lamps are essentially just large chunks of salt with a lightbulb in the middle. Pretty cutting edge. But the soft pink light they emit does create a feeling of calm and ease. You can buy one for your home or office if you so choose.

- **Do shielding techniques.** See Chapter 13.

- **Burn incense.** Smell is a powerful trigger of emotion for some people. Many people find burning incense to be very effective at calming their nerves, reducing stress, and bringing them back into a "flow" state of peace. Some incense aromas you may try for relieving stress are sandalwood, lavender, jasmine, and chamomile.

- **Take a hot bath or shower.** Nothing feels quite like a hot bath, does it? If you've had a long, stressful day at work, hop in a warm, soothing bath. Set the mood with dim lighting and maybe some music if you like. Add some Epsom salts to your bath as well to enjoy the added stress-relief benefits—anything to help you ease the tension of the day. A shower can do the same. Let the warm water put your body at ease, clearing your mind of the day's thoughts.

Plan ahead and schedule some self-care strategies for before, during, and after work. Get organized and make self-care a part of your day. Schedule it in as you would any meeting, grocery-shopping session, or Kelly Clarkson concert. These stress-management tools don't have to be for "emergency" purposes only. They can be useful tips to practice during a time you have chosen to focus on self-care.

All these ideas are aimed at releasing and managing stress in a healthy way. You want to have as many tips, tricks, and coping strategies as you can think of available to you in your stress-management tool kit. Life is dynamic and always changing. A particular stress-management tool may work for you one day but not so well the next. With all these ideas at your fingertips, pick the ones that work the best—that resonate with you in the moment. Keep thumbing through your Rolodex of ways to handle stress, and as your day changes, change up your tactics. The more tools and ideas you have, the more prepared you'll feel. Next, go to work and have confidence in managing all the stress and stimuli you face.

Now that you're centered and you know how to release stress, go enjoy that Clarkson concert!

11

Venting. It's Not Just for Dryers

My grandmother once told me when I was very young that she hated complainers, and I took that to heart. I respect the sage wisdom of my grandmother, and so, for the rest of my life I have kept my complaints to myself. "I don't want to be one of 'those' people," I'd say. Have you ever worked with someone for whom every word out of their mouth is a complaint about something? It's like they go out of their way to be unhappy about everything and they want the entire work space to be aware of it. It's annoying and exhausting listening to someone complain all day long. It's emotionally and physically draining. So, with my grand-mother's words ringing in my ears, I have always tried to keep my complaints to a minimum.

Holding in all my complaints taught me to be a problem

solver. Instead of whining about something, I would offer a solution. This made sense to me. But what it also taught me was to internalize all my anger and hostility toward those mean jerks at work. If someone pushed me around or hurt my feelings, I wouldn't say anything. I was afraid to be branded a complainer, therefore I never expressed myself. I would just let my emotions boil up inside me like a pressure cooker ready to blow. I knew this didn't feel good, but what could I do? I'm not a complainer. I have learned since, however, not to confuse venting with complaining.

I believe there is a difference between venting and complaining. Venting is a healthy form of self-expression that helps in the release of emotions. This is constructive and a helpful tool to use when you're feeling upset about someone at work. Complaining, on the other hand, is born of the mind-set that everything is the worst and that life is unfair and horrible. The act of complaining focuses on negative energy and keeps your mind occupied with exactly the thing you'd like to change, and in turn, creates more of it. *"Where your mind goes, energy flows."* Since you're reading this book and trying to change your life in a positive way, I take it you'd rather do the former than the latter.

Holding on to negative emotions is so detrimental to a person's well-being. Dwelling on a hurtful comment from a coworker and never expressing that emotion to release it from your mind, body, and spirit can create a deep well of suffering inside you. And it hurts. We end up taking that pain all over town.

A great way to let go of your pain or anger quickly is to vent to someone. Go and talk to a trusted colleague or a close friend or family member. Look for someone who will listen and hear what you have to say. You're looking for someone you feel comfortable with who makes you feel at ease. With this person, you can jettison all your frustration and anger, and feel it leaving you in an ebbing wave of relief. It feels good to get things off your chest. Try to focus on how good it feels to express yourself and let things go.

It may feel like complaining at first. But once you vent to a trusted friend, they may put a hand on your shoulder and help you feel supported. Now your feelings are validated, and this feels good! It feels good to get help. We're all in this together. Let's help each other and show compassion as often as we can.

There's a big difference between people who vent to express themselves in a constructive way and those who choose to complain and find the worst in everything. It's OK to express yourself. Your feelings are valid, and you are not alone. Find someone to talk to.

Other ideas for venting and self-expression:

- Call or text a friend.
- Video chat with someone.
- See a professional counselor or therapist.
- Start a video diary (either just for you or to share).
- Write to yourself.
- Write to a friend.
- Exercise (a physical act of venting; your body is expressing itself through movement).
- Play an instrument.
- Dance.
- Paint, draw, or make some other form of art.
- Cry.
- Do yoga.

Releasing emotion is a healthy process. Find what works for you and build a trusted group of people you can vent to when need be. It helps.

12

All about Grounding

"Yeah, what is grounding?"

Grounding is tapping into and aligning with the
vibration and energy frequency of the earth, to help
fully integrate your mind, body, and spirit into the
present moment.

This technique is groundbreaking! It is my go-to exercise
when I'm feeling anxious or panicked for any reason. It
helps calm me down and bring me to a relaxed state of
mind. The idea is that our physical bodies are part of this
world. The food we eat, the air we breathe, the water we
drink . . . it all comes from the earth. This planet is a part
of us, and we are forever connected to it. To its energy. Just
like the rock in the dirt, the trees in the forest, the waves
in the ocean. All of it is part of this crazy planet we call

home, just like we are. To be grounded means to coexist alongside all these things. To walk among nature and *be* a part of it. To feel like we all share the same energy, as if the rock, trees, waves, and we ourselves aren't these separate things but somehow . . . one. We share the same energy, and if we want to live healthy, balanced lives, we need to stay connected to it all.

When you are grounded, there is no Geiger counter or machine to show this; you just have to feel it. Your emotions are the first tell-tale sign of connectivity. Being grounded feels like you're completely aware that your body is here, in the present moment. You're very aware of feeling pulled by gravity, toward the earth. You feel happy, content, and comfortably dense and connected to the ground you're standing on. Breathing becomes easier, and there is an overwhelming sense of relaxation and security in being where you are—with your feet planted on the ground.

Feeling grounded is like having a flashlight with fresh batteries. It turns on easily, and the beam of light is steady, strong, and bright. It works well and illuminates everything around you. What happens, though, when the batteries are old? The flashlight flickers on and off, and the light becomes so dim you can barely tell it's working. You have to knock it with the palm of your hand, trying to get more electrical juice to flow to the bulb. The connection is very weak—like feeling ungrounded.

"OK, but why would I not be grounded?"

Knowing that we're a part of the energy frequency of the earth adds a baseline understanding of our overall health. When we're humming along at the same frequency as the planet, we're doing pretty well. We feel grounded. But when we get knocked off balance, become disconnected, and start vibrating at too high or too low a frequency, we can feel overwhelmed, uncomfortably light, panicked, anxious, frantic, or unfocused, and over prolonged periods, this can even lead to illness and disease. Cold feet and poor circulation are other signs of a weak connection with the earth.

We become ungrounded for various reasons, but the main one we'll talk about here is an overactive mind. We have evolved to be self-aware, to think critically and ask the big questions: *Who am I? What is the meaning of life? Why did Beanie Babies stop being popular?* Yes, the human mind has evolved a great deal in the past 10,000 years. Almost too much. It was designed to "think," so the mind says, *OK, let's do it all!* You think about real-estate prices, about the food you need to buy, about getting the car serviced, about that show you watched, about the coworker who obsesses over Jake Gyllenhaal, about losing weight, about stress and traffic and recycling and birds and babies and beer . . . The mind jumps from one thing to another with astonishing speed, like trying to set the world record for running errands in a Formula 1 race car. As it does this, the mind and the body disassociate from one another. That's not good. To be a whole and balanced person, you need your mind, body, and spirit and the earth's energy all working together. If even one is out of whack, the others will be affected.

We have basically become so evolved that we now have to actively think about something we used to do naturally—to actively be aware of the present moment. Look at bears or owls or salamanders. They don't think about stock portfolios or antidiarrheal medication. They just simply *are*. They exist in the moment, either hunting for food, looking for water, or mating. They are nature's masters at being present. We, however, have lost that bearlike natural connection with being present—with being grounded. Now, to stay grounded, we have to actively work at it. We do this by controlling the mind, getting calm and present, and then doing things that connect us with the energy of the earth.

Balancing and calming the mind allows for a calm body.

When your body is calm, you can get grounded to the earth's energy. When you live a grounded life, your mind can accept and reflect that healing energy from the earth and let it cycle back all over again. You just have to pay attention.

Some other things that may cause you to become ungrounded are anxiety and stress; confusion, panic, or feelings of being overwhelmed; consuming sugar or caffeine; movies, TV programs, or commercials that cause anxiety; and ungrounded people who try to ground themselves *through you.* Any long-term distraction that takes your attention away from being present can lead to feeling ungrounded.

How to Become More Grounded

1. **Do breathing exercises.** Sitting quietly and breathing deeply helps ground your energy. Try inhaling for a slow count of four, then exhaling to the same count. Repeat this six more times. Notice how you feel afterward. By focusing on your breathing, you gently bring your mind back to the present moment.

2. **Drink tea.** A nice, warm cup of tea can feel comforting and bring your attention to feeling calm and relaxed. In this state of being present, it's easier

to feel grounded.

3. **Meditate.** If you haven't caught on yet, meditating is a central theme in this book. Learning to meditate is one of the best ways to center yourself and ground your energy. Clear your mind and bring your attention to the *now*.

4. **Be in nature.** You know that feeling of awareness and vitality that comes with just being in nature? That's because nature is incredibly healing for us. The Japanese even have a name for it: *Shinrin-yoku*—"forest bathing."

5. **Try visualization techniques.** Sit quietly with your eyes closed and imagine a place or time when you felt grounded. Some examples could be standing on a beach watching a sunset over the ocean, sitting by the campfire at night under a sky full of stars, or walking through a beautiful green forest. Use whatever images calm and relax you and help reaffirm what the earth's energy feels like.

6. **Eat potatoes, carrots, and other root vegetables.** Nutrition plays a huge role in how you feel. Eating organic vegetables that come from the earth, especially those that grow underground, helps align your energy with the earth's frequency.

7. **Walk barefoot in the grass.** The earth has a natural,

negative electrical charge that moves easily through conductors it comes in contact with, including people. In our day-to-day, we build up electrical stress throughout our bodies that can easily be released by connecting with this naturally occurring field in the ground. Find a park or grassy area and take off your shoes. Walk around for a bit and pay attention to how you feel. Describe subtle changes in your mood and the tactile sensations you observe. Walking barefoot, connected with the earth, optimizes your immune system, reduces stress, and increases an overall sense of calm and happiness. It can even improve your sleep. According to an article published online in 2012 by the *Journal of Environmental Public Health* titled "Earthing: Health Implications of Reconnecting the Human Body to the Earth's Surface Electrons,"[1] when two groups of people were tested for sleep differences, "Most grounded subjects described symptomatic improvement, while most in the [ungrounded] control group did not."

8. **Massage your legs and feet**. A good massage

---

1 Chevalier, Gaétan, et al., "Earthing: Health Implications of Reconnecting the Human Body to the Earth's Surface Electrons," *Journal of Environmental and Public Health*, January 12, 2012, www.ncbi.nlm. nih.gov/pmc/articles/PMC3265077/.

releases tension in muscles and relieves stress. It also focuses your attention on the parts of your body that come in contact with the ground. Being conscious of where your body touches the ground helps with feeling grounded again.

9. **Have pictures that ground you.** Decorate your surroundings with photos that remind you of the outdoors, of feeling grounded. A waterfall, a sunset, a desert, the ocean, a night sky full of stars . . . these images can instill a feeling of calm and keep the mind focused on the sensations that grounding produces. This is a powerful tool.

10. **Burn incense.** Burning incense and stimulating your sense of smell can be very useful in becoming more grounded. It relaxes your mind so you can focus on feeling connected with the earth's energy. Some great ideas for grounding incense are lavender, sandalwood, and sage.

11. **Take a shower, go swimming, or just be near water.**[2] Water is a cure-all purifier. Not only does

2 Jiang, Shu-Ye, Ali Ma, and Srinivasan Ramachandran, "Negative Air Ions and Their Effects on Human Health and Air Quality Improvement," *International Journal of Molecular Sciences* 19, no. 10 (2018): 2966. http://dx.doi.org/10.3390/ijms19102966.

taking a bath remove dirt and clear the pores in your skin, but just being close to water can give you the benefits of better air quality, too. The electrical stress we accumulate washes away in the shower because the shearing force of water releases negative ions (oxygen atoms with an extra electron), which attach to and neutralize positive ions that build up from the body and in the air. This helps clean the air of particulates so you can breathe better. This also explains why we feel a greater sense of well-being and improved mood during rainstorms or when we're at the beach or near a waterfall or mountain stream.

12. **Read a book or watch a movie.** Reading a good book is a great way to focus your mind, let go of overthinking, and just be present so you feel still and more grounded. The same can be said for a comforting movie. When you have time, sit down and watch a movie that promotes good feeling vibes, calms you down, and leaves you feeling aware of the present moment. Be mindful that you don't watch too much TV, though. Remember, prolonged distractions of any sort lead to detachment from the earth's energy. Watching a good movie is a grounding tool, not a lifestyle.

13. **Exercise.** Getting just 20 minutes of exercise is a

great way to release energetic resistance, center your attention, and become more grounded. Sign up for a gym membership or buy a pair of running shoes and start exercising. Finding ways to keep active gets your blood and energy flowing and makes it easier to feel the effects of grounding.

14. **Start gardening.** Buy some flowers and get digging! Gardening is good for grounding because it's a calm, slow activity in which you're physically touching and working with the earth. Get your hands dirty and see if you experience a heightened sense of fulfillment, improved mood, and overall well-being.

15. **Listen to grounding music.** Tones and music can have a major influence on your connectivity to the earth's energy. Try experimenting with Tibetan singing bowls for a different kind of meditation or listen to calming music that moves you. Anything that focuses your attention on the present moment and actively helps you feel connected to the earth will help.

16. **Practice yoga or tai chi.**[3] Yoga and tai chi have

---

3 Harvard Health Publishing, "The Health Benefits of Tai Chi," *Harvard Health*, May 2009, www.health.harvard.edu/staying-healthy/the-health-benefits-of-tai-chi.

grown in popularity for helping to promote stronger muscles, better fitness, and improved mood. But in terms of energy, what's happening when you practice these disciplines is that your chi (your spirit) and your awareness are coming into balance, too. In Chinese philosophy it is said that chi is an energy force that flows through the body. Exercising and moving the body helps to remove energy blockages and promote overall health. These practices are great for grounding!

Try these two grounding meditations.

1. **Imagine roots of trees.** Sit in a comfortable, quiet place where you can breathe and get calm. Breathe in and out for a few minutes while you settle yourself into the moment. Just bring your attention to your breath. When any thoughts or ideas crop up, acknowledge them and let them pass. Once you've become calm, begin to visualize a wonderful forest full of tall redwood trees, green leaves, and spongy, leaf-laden ground beneath your bare feet. As you walk, gently stepping on the soft ground, you make your way to

the largest tree in the forest. You approach slowly, with respect, and ask Spirit to help ground your energy. Standing now at the base of the tree, reach out with your mind and place a hand on the trunk. Imagine all the roots underground, reaching deep into the earth. This tree is permanently connected with the earth, and by touching it, you too feel grounded. You can feel the energy of the planet resonating through the roots, your feet, your whole body, in all things around you. Feel this connection in nature and bring it with you, through your day.

2. **Imagine an anchor.** After you've spent a few moments meditating and getting calm, try this visualization. Imagine you're standing in a field of tall grass up to your knees. It's a beautiful day with blue skies, snowcapped mountains in the background, and purple flowers scattered in all directions. You take a few slow steps and feel the grass caress your skin as you begin to explore this world. Now take a moment, stand still, and imagine an anchor with a heavy chain made of white light attached to your lower back, at your tailbone. Pretend this chain leads straight into the ground, to the center of the earth. And here your anchor lies, pulling gently at the center

of the planet. Feel this connection. When the earth spins, you spin with it. When the sun rises to warm the earth, it warms your body, too. You are connected through this lifeline at any time you wish to feel it. You are grounded. You are a part of Earth, and it is a part of you.

In addition: Some grounding techniques I have pursued are considered alternative medicine or pseudoscience. They helped tremendously, though, and I still enjoy learning about new ideas for healing and grounding. For example, you may carry hematite in your pocket. Hematite is a stone and a primary ore of iron. It is silver and metallic looking and is dense in weight. Having a small piece of hematite with you at work can influence your energy field and help get you grounded. Also, study your chakra system and learn to balance all seven energy hotspots in your body. Your first chakra, or root chakra, is located at the base of your spine and is the seat of grounding and a sense of connectivity to the earth. For more info on energy medicine, check out *Intuition Medicine: The Science of Energy*, by Francesca McCartney.

This is definitely not an exhaustive list of grounding tips. Do your homework and don't be afraid to try new things.

Pay attention to what works best for you and make these tricks part of your daily life.

13.

All about Shielding

"Right, so, *shielding*. What is it? Why is it important? How can it help empaths at work?"

Shielding is a technique by which you protect yourself from all the overwhelming energy around you. The idea is that with an energetic guard surrounding your body, you become less susceptible to the stressors in your environment—like how a raincoat keeps you dry. This is important for empaths because it helps to deflect negative energy and keep you feeling safe.

Empaths don't just feel the energy and emotions of others. We absorb them and take them in as our own. Our energy field is naturally open and accommodating, like a beachfront hotel lobby in Hawaii—everyone is free to come and go. This is why sensitive people get exhausted so easily. It's a lot to process. We're constantly having to deal with new energies, all day, every day. That many stimuli can be overwhelming. Without a mindfulness practice in place, we freely absorb all this energy, and it is very draining.

Have you ever been on a train and looked out the window? Some people sit quietly and let the nearby, passing scenery blur together in one continuous blend of hazy obscurity. They don't focus or latch onto anything but instead let all the trees, traffic, and buildings distort into one. But for an empath, life is like letting your eyes dart rapidly from object to object, trying to focus and understand every . . . single . . . passing . . . detail. That's how it is with our energy field, too. We have a very hard time separating ourselves from the landscape. We try to observe, process, understand, and relate every form of stimulus available, and it's exhausting.

Shielding can help with this. There are a few methods of protecting your energy field so you don't absorb so much information out in the world. Let's go over some of them now.

Shielding Techniques

1. **Visualization.** Find a quiet, safe place where you can be alone. Sit down, take some deep breaths, and empty

your mind. Meditate for a few moments and get relaxed. When you're ready, begin with a full body scan.

Close your eyes and feel your body. Feel present. Really pay attention to the act of breathing, in and out. Start going throughout your whole body and observing how each part of your body feels. Notice any sensations and describe them to yourself. The muscles in your feet. The weight of your shoulders. The tingling in your hands and fingers. The pressure in your stomach. Notice anything at all, breathe, and let it go. The point of this full-body mindfulness practice is to get you tuned in and paying attention to the present moment and your being in it. In the *now*. When your mind is calm and relaxed, your body can relax and fall back into its natural state of calm. Now that you're aware of how your body is meant to feel, you can get better at protecting it.

With your eyes closed, begin to imagine a bright light forming around your body. It can be a brilliant white light. Or maybe a warm yellowish orange. Or even a vivid purple. What color you feel most comfortable with is up to you. You're looking for a calm, safe color.

This light starts slowly at first, becoming brighter and brighter with every breath you take. The more you breathe, the brighter and stronger it gets. This is your shield. Imagine that it is as strong as steel. Hard as diamonds. Nothing can penetrate this shield. You are completely safe.

Your shield can be the shape of your body. It can be a bubble, a dome, or a pyramid. Pick a shape and size that resonates with you. I change the size, shape, and color of my shield often, just to try new ones. But my favorites are a translucent purple dome the size of a house and a sunset-colored, body-shaped shield that I carry around like a cocoon. It all depends on what resonates with me in the moment. I go with what feels right.

Keep breathing steadily and mindfully. Your shield is growing stronger and more brilliant now. Imagine that within this shield, you feel protected. You feel such a great sense of safety, such an overwhelming sense of protection and security, that nothing can touch you. In this force field you've created, you are at your most calm and in your most relaxed natural state.

This shield is like a barrier that nothing can cross. Imagine watching particles of energy trying to enter your shield, but bounce off. You're completely focused within your protected shield and paying attention to this calm you've created. As you do, all the energy of your environment is moving around, bouncing and gliding off your shield. Nothing is getting in.

Now you can smile. You are safe. You are protected. Your shield is strong.

Open your eyes and feel this fantastic sense of strength and confidence you've created. Be mindful of this shield and imagine it is with you. Take this shield with you to work and keep it close. Anytime you become distracted from this calm state, acknowledge it and find time to bring your mind back to your shield.

The more you practice mindfully walking around with your shield, the easier it becomes.

2. **Shielding stones and crystal energy.** Another method of shielding yourself at work is to carry stones or crystals with you. There is a popular belief in alternative medicine that minerals have metaphysical properties that can channel healing energy. Some rocks or crystals are thought to have shielding properties that can deter unwanted negative energy so you don't absorb it into your body. You can carry small stones in your pocket, wear them as jewelry, or keep some at work, in your car, and at home. Some shielding stones to consider are obsidian, black tourmaline, and amethyst.

Although there is limited scientific data to confirm the healing powers of crystals, it's more important, I think, to see how you feel when you interact with various minerals. **Trust your emotions.** Do some research and head to your nearest crystal shop to learn more. See if this shielding technique is for you. You can also search online by typing:

Shielding stones for empaths
Crystal shop near me
New Age shop
Metaphysical properties of gemstones

3. **A good offense.** The best defense is a good offense— meaning, in this case, that when you feel good and you're focused on positivity, you're not a vibrational match for negativity. Exude as much positive energy as you can. This is a shield, too, and a strong one at that. Strive to be at work already feeling so good, so fulfilled, and so excited to be alive that nothing bothers you. Become a master at focusing your mind on feeling good and building your inner strength. As you do so, negative energy will part around you like a stream around a rock. Like a shield.

Walk into work like a rock star.
Then nothing can touch you.

We have spoken about creating joy from within and living an unconditional life. Put some time and effort into this practice and it will improve your life in so many ways. Get to that good feeling place often, and when you have to go to work, moonwalk into the office and blast Katy Perry on your phone! Get excited and show the world how great you feel. You're telling the universe, "Hey, I feel great today! I love myself, and things are working out for me!" By giving love, you receive it in return. The pain and negativity you're used to will begin to fade away.

I like to imagine that I have no shield. My barrier is down and I'm open to all the energy around me. But this time, I feel so abundant, so clear and powerful, that it all just zips around me. All the energy I used to absorb like a sponge is still there, I can still feel it, but I let it pass through me. I become this transparent, nonphysical being, like the wind. I let all the negative energy just go right by, and I retain only the emotions that I choose to feel, like love and joy. No more resisting. Just being. Just allowing.

Imagine that you're a rock sitting in a stream. The

constant bombardment of stimuli and energy in your day is here, front and center, flowing like the water. Coming at you from all directions. But you are like the rock, unmoved and unimpressed by this free-flowing noise. All this energy flows around you, smooth around your curves, and continues downstream. You have no shield to guard against the stream, but today you don't need it. You are like the rock, strong and unbreakable. Nothing can touch you. You decide how to be.

Summary: At the end of the day, the more energy-management tools you have in your tool box, the better. Having a shield is a great technique for protecting your energy. But I suggest focusing the bulk of your long-term efforts on building inner strength, feeling love, and getting to that good feeling place. That's where you'll find the infinite power inside you.

14

How to Set Boundaries

What is setting boundaries? *It is identifying personal limits and your comfort level and expressing those limits to others.*

Setting boundaries is such an important life skill for an empath or highly sensitive person. It will enable you to say yes and no when you feel like it. For many people this is a no-brainer, but for the few, the proud, the empaths/ HSPs of the world, we struggle with saying no because we want to please people and make them happy. We tend to say yes to everyone.

Learning to set healthy boundaries is about knowing yourself and what you're comfortable with. It's about protecting your energy and emotions from unhealthy or unwanted situations in life. This is an especially important skill for an empath because we get overwhelmed and exhausted by the energy around us. We must be doubly mindful of how we feel so we can enforce those boundaries and practice the self-care we deserve. Without good boundaries, we become subject to all manner of toxic energy.

Ways to Set Boundaries

This skill is applicable in other areas of your life, but let's focus on work. To get started, identify situations that tend to make you feel uncomfortable, off balance, unhappy, or resentful. Think about what you wish you could have said before this situation occurred. How would you have handled things differently? Setting healthy boundaries enables you to speak up and express how you feel about something. This means letting other people know what you think. This can be a scary prospect if you're new to voicing how you feel, but it gets easier with practice.

If you know working 10 hours a day is too much for you, alter your schedule and work less, if possible.

If you feel pressured to attend a party but don't want to stay all night, go for a comfortable period of time, then politely say your good-byes and head home.

If someone asks you to help them move, but you're not feeling well, say no.

If a friend uses you like a therapist on whom to dump all their emotional stress and it feels like way too much, tell them. A good friend will understand.

If you're at the dinner table with your family and you're not comfortable with the food being served, be polite and ask for an alternative. Stick with salad, or anticipate this and eat beforehand. Assert your needs.

"No" is a complete sentence.

Setting boundaries isn't complicated. It's knowing where you feel safe and comfortable and making decisions based on maintaining that feeling. Practicing this, especially if you have been saying yes to people for so many years, can feel like driving a new car for the first time. It may feel weird, and people may seem put off by the new you, or even a little hurt or jealous. But it feels amazing to make a change that honors the new you.

Set your intention to stand up for yourself. Voice how you feel.

Affirmations for getting comfortable with setting boundaries:

- I don't have to say yes to everything.
- I know my limits.
- "No" is a complete sentence.

- It is OK to say no.
- It feels good to express myself.
- People accept and approve of how I feel.
- Setting boundaries feels good.

If someone asks you for something, take some time to think about it before you commit to an answer. It is easy for a sensitive person to say yes in the moment without thinking. It's a reflex to say yes all the time, thinking that it will make people like you or that you're putting other people's needs before yours. Be mindful and tactful in your responses when speaking to people at work and in general. If you need to think about your answer, tell them you'll get back to them later. This is totally acceptable.

Think about your workplace and a time when you agreed to do something and later felt resentful. Have you agreed to stay late at work to be nice, then wished you had just gone home? Do people expect you to volunteer for things, and then you do and feel totally overwhelmed? It's OK to put yourself first and express your boundaries.

Examples of boundary setting:
- "Sorry, I can't stay late tonight."
- "I'm not going to plan the holiday party this year. I'm

not feeling up to it."

- "I can't make it to the movies like we planned. Can we reschedule?"
- "I'm feeling tired. I think I'm going to head home."
- "Excuse me, could you please speak a little more softly? I have very sensitive hearing."

When voicing how you feel, get comfortable being honest with people. You shouldn't feel the need to come up with excuses for why you're saying no. No is enough. And if someone asks, just say you're not comfortable with whatever it is, or not feeling up to it. You don't need an alibi or a way to circumvent the truth to make people accept your boundaries. You know where you're comfortable, and that's your priority. You're not worried about whether people like your boundaries. Instead, you're secure and stable in knowing who you are.

Just breathe. Speak up and out and express how you feel about things. Your friends will love and respect your boundaries, and for the people who don't? Well . . . we're not concerned with them anyway. So the next time a situation pops up at work that threatens your personal boundaries, a bell should go off in your head. This is the perfect opportunity to practice saying no.

If you are ready to set boundaries but need some help asserting yourself, turn the page.

15

How to Be Assertive

One of the most obvious but commonly overlooked techniques for dealing with coworkers is talking to them. Simply communicating and asserting how you feel to a coworker, however, often isn't even a consideration for a sensitive, introverted person, as we sidestep conflict at every turn. This chapter will teach you how to stand up for yourself and communicate your needs.

Highly sensitive people and empaths have a notoriously hard time speaking up and asserting themselves. We are extremely sensitive to conflict and prefer to remain passive in all matters. We shy away from asserting our needs. We fear being judged for our beliefs, or contradicted or criticized. The thought of someone disagreeing and our then having to deal with that opposing energy sounds uncomfortable and panic inducing—*better to stay in shallow waters, where it is safe.* Which is why you rarely hear a strong opinion from an empath/ HSP . . . on anything! *What if someone doesn't like what I have to say?* So we keep quiet for the most part, preferring to be the peacekeepers of the work environment.

But in this silence we lose something special. It's as if we are putting a finger over the mouth of our inner voice, hushing it and telling it not to make a sound. This restrictive behavior squelches your inner spirit, the inner you, and constricts the need to feel free, outspoken, and alive. We all deserve to feel true to our nature, confident in our beliefs and living fulfilled lives—lives in which we're free to express ourselves. *Doesn't that rock?*

It can be scary as heck, though, speaking up for the first time. You may feel completely paralyzed by fear and panic at the thought of voicing how you feel. That's OK. There are three easy steps to becoming an assertive wizard. Ready?

1. Practice.

2. Practice.

3. Practice.

All it takes for you to become a more assertive, outspoken individual is to practice. Treat being assertive as you would any other skill, like playing the violin or building a rocket ship. If you want to get good at something, you have to practice.

It's a bummer that some people do this assertive thing so naturally, while empaths and HSPs have to take deep breaths and practice a hundred times before asking someone to turn their music down.

1. To get started, practice at home or wherever else you feel safe. Find a spot to sit and relax and go over the events of the day. How was work? What did you do? Try to pinpoint some times today when you could have spoken up and said something; when you could have voiced your opinion.

   Start with something small, like "I could have corrected that barista for getting my order wrong" or "I could have totally joined that conversation today about *The Office*. I watch that show, too." Easy stuff. It doesn't have to be controversial. It shouldn't be at first. Don't dive into the deep end and interrupt a safety meeting with "Here's what I think about religion and politics!" Yeah, please don't do that.

2. Next, imagine going back through your day and actually asserting yourself in those scenarios. Really home in and focus on what you would say. How would you say it? What do you think their reaction would be?

Imagine a positive reaction from your coworkers, and your input being well received.

This little exercise is to get you thinking about small ways to begin asserting what you think in the workplace. Practice on your own. Imagine standing up for yourself until you feel comfortable going to the next step.

3. Finally, let's put it into practice.

HOMEWORK

Now that you've practiced what to say on your own, let's try it out on a day when you're going to work. You will see that same coworker who causes you trouble. Before you head to work, say, "Today, I am going to find one instance in which to speak up for myself. I am going to find a way to say what I mean and how I feel. Just one time. I can do this." After you've made this commitment, go to work and get busy looking for ways to assert yourself. Keep your eyes open for any opportunity, no matter how small, to speak up and out. You can do it!

Example: You're riding in the car with your difficult coworker and they are listening to that radio station you hate. Deep breath . . . "Hey, could we listen to something else?"

Example: You overhear a conversation at lunch in which some coworkers say they like spicy food, and others don't. Join in. Speak up and say, "Hey, I like spicy food."

Example: You're about to watch a long-winded presentation and your boss says, "Does anyone need to use the restroom before we get started?" No one raises their hand, because no one wants to be "that" person. But if ya gotta go, say something! Raise that hand high! There will be others who are glad you did.

After your first triumph at work, ask yourself, *How'd it go?* Was it as bad as you thought it would be? Or did asserting your opinion turn out to be no big deal? No matter how it was received by your coworkers, go out and celebrate. You were assertive today! Do your happy dance and mock-sing "We Are the Champions" into your TV remote, because today you rocked it!

Extra Credit: If you're gathering steam, becoming a master at asserting yourself, and need a challenge, put this book down, stand, and shout for the whole world to hear . . . "I AM BEAUTIFUL, AMAZING, AND WORTHY!" Wasn't that fun?

"Am I being assertive or aggressive?"

Maybe it's an empath/ HSP thing. Or perhaps it's my midwestern manner, but I have always had a hard time standing up for myself. I think I have always associated mean people with loud, arrogant, outspoken individuals who don't care about anyone. All the ill-tempered colleagues I've worked with over the years seem to have shared similar qualities. They tend to have big voices and big opinions, enjoy confrontation, love being the center of attention, and show little regard for the feelings of others. Since I definitely did not want to be like that (mean or coldhearted), my mind made the connection that this meant not being loud or outspoken, either.

I have always considered myself to be a nice person, and by staying quiet and reserved, I avoided replicating any of those characteristics I find repugnant in the mean people of the world. Unfortunately, by steering clear of being loud and having a voice, I also lost the ability to assert myself. And that's no way to be. I wanted to speak up, but I was afraid of being perceived as a loud, obnoxious jerk.

It took me a long time to understand that there is a difference between being assertive and being aggressive. Aggressive people are always on guard, ready for a fight. They are looking for confrontation and for ways to assert their opinions and dominance over others. Aggressive is yelling. Aggressive is hurtful and puts people down. Assertive, however, is different.

Being assertive means voicing how you feel in a clear, direct fashion—speaking your mind openly, using upfront communication. You can be forceful without yelling. You can express strong emotions without berating someone. Being assertive is using strong, deliberate speech to get your point across. And speaking your mind and expressing your feelings, especially for an empath/ HSP, is necessary for a healthy, balanced state of being. Without feeling able to express yourself and assert your needs, you can become a pushover at work. Your voice is constricted. Your emotions become bottlenecked, trapped within you and causing problems.

It's OK to be assertive and have your voice be heard. Don't be afraid of coming off as mean. It can feel that way at first, especially if you're new to asserting how you feel. But keep at it. Pay attention to how it feels after you voice your opinion. It can feel so good to express yourself and release blocked emotions, simply by letting other people know where you stand. Additionally, remember that you're an empath/ HSP with unique gifts. You recognize and consider the feelings of others. There's less of a chance of your being overly aggressive because you'll feel it immediately if you've pissed someone off. You got this.

It can be frightening at first and may make you feel way out of your comfort zone. That's OK. Being assertive takes practice, but over time, it gets easier and feels more natural. Soon, you may find that you comfortably speak up for yourself all the time. You're becoming that strong, confident version of yourself you always imagined you could be.

16

Imagine Being Awesome

One of the greatest tools I've learned for dealing with stress and evil coworkers is visualizing a better scenario. I imagine a life where everything at work goes my way and life is easy. The people at work treat me with respect and give me compliments all day. They are supportive and understanding, and going to work is a fulfilling experience. But why stop there? I imagine getting a pay raise for no reason, or maybe I finally muster the courage to ask out that woman I've been interested in, and she says yes. This stuff can happen!

By imagining a better reality at work and with your coworkers, you familiarize yourself with the emotions you'd prefer to feel. Through this technique of visualizing your preferred reality, you can learn these better-feeling emotions so well that you take them to work with you. It starts to become a habit to feel this way, and in doing so, you begin to live unconditionally in your environment. You have created joy and happiness within you. And ultimately, this is how to effect a change in your work space anyhow, right? Remember, "where your mind goes, energy flows." So get happy first, and then your reality can change. Using your imagination is a powerful tool for change. To begin, when you're at home, in a quiet space, sit down, close your eyes, and imagine the perfect version of yourself.

In your imagination, where do you go? What do you want? Whom do you spend your time with? Imagine your ideal life and the perfect you. The most important part of this exercise isn't the specifics of what you want, but how it makes you *feel*. The emotion. Describe these emotions to yourself in great detail using as many adjectives as you can.

Examples: *Now that I am the perfect version of myself, I feel joyful. Relaxed. Easy. Peaceful. Quiet. Fun. Full of laughter. Fulfilled. Abundant. Uplifted. Excited! Focus your attention on these words and others that come to you and how they make you feel.*

This is a powerful method of effecting change in every aspect of your life, but specifically with coworkers. It's helpful to begin with your ideal situation at work. Still sitting quietly, use your imagination and pretend that that awful coworker you deal with every day is now super-friendly and compassionate. This person is helpful, polite, apologetic, and diligent in their work and fosters a sense of harmony around the workplace. Now ask yourself, how does this make you feel? Does this feel like an improvement? Do you feel more relaxed? At ease? Can you breathe a little easier? Is your work space more joyful now that this person isn't a drag? Again, describe these emotions to yourself in great detail and focus on them as you finish this visualization practice.

Now that you have identified your preferred reality and the good emotions associated with it—*good like a glass of red wine in a hot tub overlooking St. Lucia good*—let's put it into practice. Let's go to work.

Keep using your imagination, living in this headspace of peaceful tranquillity, and go to work, where it is likely to be the same old routine. Work is the same stressful place with the same people you left yesterday. The same behavior and bothersome conversations are still present, only this time, you feel different. You're watching the scene at work as an objective observer. You see what is happening, but you don't attach any bias, emotion, or meaning behind it. Maybe that irksome coworker is being a knucklehead again, in your face and fired up about something irrelevant. Be a part of the conversation as much as needed, but keep your emotions in that good feeling place you practiced before you arrived. Your focus is still on how you'd prefer to feel. Take a deep breath and smile, because you'll start to notice that this coworker bothers you less and less. This person or situation at work can't affect you, because so much of your attention is on those good feelings you practiced earlier. While you may be at work, getting tasks done, your energy and emotions are all feeling good, happy, and buoyant. Living an unconditional life feels great!

Example: You have been practicing using your imagination to create a more ideal work environment, and it feels good. It feels good to focus on relief, ease, peace, fun, and fulfillment. It is Tuesday morning now, and you just arrived at work.

You walk through the front door, and you notice all the same things you're used to: the broken vending machine, the coffee brewing, and the low hum of electricity flowing through lights, computers, and air-conditioning. As you make your way to your desk, out of your peripheral vision you see that one person, that coworker you're dreading having to talk to. And your heart skips and beats a little harder, thudding deeply in your chest.

But wait. You catch yourself and acknowledge this misstep in the focused mindfulness you've been practicing. Ah, that's right. I love feeling at ease and relaxed and happy and full of compassion. This feels so much better. How silly to get anxious at the sight of someone. *And thus you bring your mind back to that good feeling place.*

You start to get set for the day, and suddenly, there is that person—a devil dressed in business-casual, Kohl's attire. (Or overalls, depending on where you work. Heck, maybe they're a florist wearing a Deadpool T-shirt.)

While they start talking and you feel a well of panic threaten to overtake your mind, you breathe deeply again, reminding yourself of the emotions you love. Bring your thoughts back to your preferred good feeling place. (The mind loves to wander and get distracted, doesn't it? Like a child in a museum being told not to touch anything.)

This coworker is still talking, and you're listening, but at the same time, you're emotionally swimming in the waters of your own private seaside pool. You notice the same twinge of anger and pain inside you, wanting, begging for attention, because this person has caused you so much stress in the past. But you're an observer today. You see your panic within you, and instead of latching on to it and letting it control you, you simply see it and say hello.

Hello, pain. Hello, suffering. I see you and acknowledge you. I deeply love and accept myself. I am choosing to feel good today. All my focus is on how great I'd prefer to feel.

Your attention comes back now to this coworker in front of you. As the conversation ends and they walk away, maintain your focus on your good feeling place. You slowly turn around and get back to what you were doing, but you notice you feel so good. Damn good, even. This person had little effect on how you feel today. You congratulate yourself, eat a cookie, and get back to it.

You have just displayed a fine example of being unconditionally happy, despite your surroundings. This is so great and a huge leap forward! Air high five!

Summary: The idea is to keep practicing how you'd prefer to feel. Practice at home, at work, in the car, out to eat . . . everywhere. And keep putting it into practice especially with the things that throw you off your game, like mean people at work. Practice this so much that it becomes habit. With time and patience, you'll develop a new way of looking at the world and dealing with people. This practice can be hard at first, and you never stop working on it. Be kind and patient with yourself; it takes time to change old habits. Eventually, though, you'll become this kickass version of yourself you never thought possible. *And you like the new you. You look damn good.*

17

Let Out Your Inner Lion So People Will Hear Its Mighty Roar

This is a fun tip to use at work to help deal with coworkers: Talk about yourself!

This chapter is aimed toward those quiet and reserved individuals who, like me, are more comfortable in silence. We don't talk unnecessarily or start many conversations. So when someone comes to chat, often they run the conversation, and we barely get a word in.

If you want to grow your confidence level and become a stronger, more independent version of yourself, practice talking about *you*. Find ways to let out your personality. When you're in a conversation at work, find a moment to express who you are as an individual.

Talking about yourself does a few things:

1. When you're talking about yourself and your interests, your bonehead coworker isn't talking about themselves for once. What a nice change of pace! Now you're not getting bogged down and drained by their incessant goings-on about irrelevant nonsense.

2. If you talk about yourself, a narcissist will recognize that you're no longer an easy target to lean on for attention. They're looking for someone to listen to them, not the other way around. These coworkers will back off and bother you less.

3. Great things could happen! Once you start talking about yourself and expressing your interests to your coworkers, you might discover someone else with the same interests. Bam! You made a new friend.

4. Lastly, talking about your interests at work puts you in a more positive frame of mind. Remember, our attitude in life really depends on what we choose to think about. If you're busy thinking, discussing, and chatting about things you love to do, guess where your mind is? It's focused on those things that bring you joy. Spending more time talking about things you love will help boost your mood and create more joy in your life. It will also help improve your confidence overall.

So, tell your coworkers about that cat you adopted. Send them an e-vite to your improv class. Wear your *Star Trek* suspenders to work. Practice that Donald Duck impression you've been working on. Get weird with it! Share your weird with others. You'll be delighted to find most of the rest of us are weird, too.

Share your personality with your coworkers, and be proud of yourself and who you are. Feel confident in your interests. If you're afraid to express yourself for fear of being judged, don't sweat it. You're not focused on *What if people judge me?* You're too busy feeling loved and supported by the people who *get* you.

Voicing your opinions and interests for the first time can be daunting, though, I know. Review the chapter about asserting yourself, keep practicing, and take it one day at a time.

"But won't I come off as one of those people who only talk about themselves? I don't want to sound conceited." No worries. Narcissists care only about themselves, and when they speak, everything out of their mouths is about them. When they talk, it's constant and only to get attention in a negative way. It's as if they've blocked your path and are forcing you to listen. They don't care what they're spouting, as long as you're giving them attention.

On the other hand, when a sensitive, caring, compassionate person talks about themselves, it's to express who they truly are. It comes from a positive place full of things that really matter. An empath talks about themselves to show the world how beautiful and unique they've become. They want to share their passions with others. It's important for the sensitive person to share these interests with someone who is genuinely listening.

That's a key difference between an empath and a narcissist. The empath needs genuine engagement when they talk about themselves. They crave deep, meaningful conversation. The narcissist doesn't care about being authentic; they typically want only face-value attention. They could talk to a concrete block with a face painted on it.

Summary: The purpose of letting your personality out at work is simple. It's a stronger, better-feeling emotion than letting a coworker talk over you. Don't be the person who just "deals with" people at work. Actively work to improve your relationships with them by showing them you're strong, confident, and good at dancing. Or whatever. You can do this!

18

Schedule Yourself Some Fun

Here's a quick tip to get you through the day. **Have something to look forward to after work**. If you're in a job that is completely awful in every way and the thought of going causes enough stress and anxiety to fill Jupiter (or some other gas giant), then this tip may be of benefit.

Getting through the workday can be so hard—especially when in every corner of the workplace we're reminded of how much we hate being there. So, instead of thinking about how painful it is to be at work, focus your mind on how excited you are to watch *Battlestar Galactica* and eat mac and cheese when you get home. (Or whatever floats your boat.) Get joyful and feel exhilarated that once the workday is done, you'll be free to do something you enjoy.

Some examples:
- When you get home, cook a delicious dinner, or start

a slow-cooker in the morning so the meal is waiting for you.

- Watch a few more episodes of that Netflix show you like.
- Go out for a drink or dinner with someone close to you.
- Hit the gym after work and get some good exercise before going home.
- Enjoy your weekly rock-climbing class or book club.
- Touch up that painting you've been working on.

By spending the day looking forward to having fun after work, you're choosing better-feeling emotions. This helps put your mind and energy in that good feeling place. And you may find that this helps make the day much more tolerable. No longer is your mind lingering on that pile of sheet metal you have to turn into dog bowls at your factory job; you're thinking about that deep-dish pizza and the new movie you're going to rent tonight. (Actually, if you bend sheet metal for a living, you may want to pay attention to that. Or next you'll be trying to distract your thoughts from a smashed thumb or something.)

If you find that you don't have anything to look forward to, start small. Make a list of things you like doing and spend some time after work doing them. Do you like sitting quietly with a cup of tea? Are you a video gamer? Do you love nature and hiking? Setting aside time to do things we enjoy is so important to our health and happiness. Practice this as much as possible. After a while, your schedule might be so full of fun things that even when you're at work, your thoughts and emotions are on all the great things you have happening in your life. Now that you are so preoccupied with enjoying life, you don't have time to think about how much you hate work. You're living an unconditional life—where happiness and feeling good are your primary vibes.

Go ahead and sign up for that acting class. Join the *Walking Dead* fan club on Meetup and go out dressed as zombies with your new friends. Learn a new language. Take tai chi lessons. Buy a fish and name it Rupert. Do things you enjoy. Often. Get busy living and think about those fun things when you're at work. Plan this stuff ahead of time so you have things to look forward to. This makes the day much more tolerable because you're thinking about something positive. And we all have the ability to choose what we think about. Choose good thoughts and have fun.

19

Getting Everyone to Like You

Work sucks. You don't have to tell me. But it becomes even tougher when you try to please everyone all the time. Why do some of us do this?

I believe it has to do with acceptance and feeling happy. For many people, our happiness and self-worth is dependent on whether people like us. If people like us, then we can feel a sense of acceptance, which feels like a form of love. It's a good feeling, being loved. At the end of the day, we're all looking for the same thing, right? To love and be loved. But when our emotional strength becomes dependent on any source other than ourselves, we give our power away. We deny the infinite well of creativity and joy from within and replace it with a subpar, short-term acceptance we feel from getting people to like us.

Aside from the common empath/ HSP need to create peace and harmony in their environment by being the peacekeeper and not rocking the boat, there are other explanations for why we seek approval from others. For example, as babies, we learned that if we were well behaved, our parents rewarded that behavior with love and affection . . . maybe a Snickers. But if we cried in public, we were reprimanded and punished. Think about being born into this world knowing nothing of the social construct in which you suddenly find yourself. What's one of the first things you learn? *If I cry, I get yelled at. If I hold back my emotions, I'm rewarded.* You're learning not only to stifle your flow of self-expression, but also to look for approval and acceptance from outside yourself: from your parents. This conditioning becomes a learned behavior that we take into adulthood—into the workplace.

This society we have created is one based on restrictive rules that define what is acceptable behavior. These rules are designed by the ego to help protect the identity and tribal "norms" of society. Remember, the ego wants to feel special, but it also wants to fit in. It wants structure and needs life to make sense. It needs to have everything in neat little rows for it to feel secure. So if you follow the rules, you can be a good drone, fall in line, and be admitted beyond the velvet rope. Any behavior outside the norm is considered unacceptable and a threat to the agreed-upon identity of society, so in turn you'll be shunned by your family, your friends, your coworkers. No more approval. No more love. So of course we want people to like us. Our very sense of safety and self-worth depends on it!

It's time, though, to take our power back. The joy and self-love we can create within us is limitless and more powerful than any halfhearted nod of approval from any source outside ourselves. Practice self-love first, and those you love will love you all the more. Follow the flow of energy. If you feel loved, then others will love you. If you like yourself, the people who matter will follow.

Ultimately, we have no control over how other people treat us. It's time to let go of trying to please everyone and get busy loving yourself. Wouldn't it be better if you could feel happiness and acceptance any old time you wish? Doesn't that sound nice? Almost makes you want to skateboard!

Recognizing that you're a people pleaser and that you need everyone to like you is the first step. Acting to effect change and take your happiness into your own hands, that's step two.

You don't "need" people to like you. It's nice to get

along with others and make friends, but if there is someone at work who is terrible to you, stop trying to win them over. They have made the decision to be a miserable person, so let it go.

It's odd. I typically get along with everyone, so in instances when a coworker is being a jerk-face, I habitually go above and beyond to console, understand, and apologize to them. I've tried getting to know them, offering support—heck, I have even done some of their work! (What's wrong with me?)

We give and we give, in the hope that we'll see the same level of compassion in return. Most people, however, are incapable of giving love and support to the same degree as an empath/ HSP can. (Especially Jerry, who never considers holding the elevator door for you, but you've helped him move apartments two times already. And he promised there'd be pizza, but there never was. Where's my pizza, Jerry?)

It's disappointing, and it hurts, but we keep trying, hoping for the best—constantly seeking some sort of validation. All this is an ill-fated attempt to win people over. Working harder to get someone to like us has never worked. Not really. So we have to learn to let it go.

How to let go of seeking outside approval:

- Acknowledge that you can't control other people's behavior. Stop worrying about what you can't control.
- Become unconditionally happy and create joy within yourself. Do this by focusing on positive thoughts and emotions that make you feel good. Now, you are no longer dependent on the approval of others to feel good about yourself.
- Spend more time and attention on the people in your life who are true, sincere friends. Their love and support is unconditional.
- Become assertive and more confident in yourself and stand by your opinions. Being true to yourself feels better than having everyone like you.

"OK, I don't care if they like me, but I can't stop worrying about what people think."
It's the same idea. You have to learn to let this go.

If you're worried about what other people think of you, you're putting their happiness before yours. You are focused on their wants. Their needs. Their Steven Seagal DVD collection. You are still trying to accommodate them and vying for their approval in some way. Let this go.

"So, what can I do?"

Well, for starters, have you ever observed those people who seemingly don't give two turtle sh-s about what other people think? They have their head held high, with a ton of unearned confidence, grinning like a billboard ad for Invisalign. As an empathic person, I have always been in awe of these people. I mean, how do they do it? They don't care what anyone thinks! They just seem to do and say whatever they want, completely unconcerned about how it makes people feel. Wow. Is it confidence, arrogance, or just ignorance?

Here is what I recommend that you, the sensitive person, do to attain a similar level of "don't give a f---" swagger: Start being selfish! That's right. I said it. Start thinking about yourself for once. It's the crux of the sensitive person to neglect themselves while always observing others, but for a change, you do you. Think about what you want. How do you want to feel today? Where do you want to eat? What playlist shall you listen to while you work? Focus your mind on how you feel and let go of what other people are doing. This will start to shift you into a very important mind-set that we keep coming back to—being mindful and practicing self-care.

It may seem as if you're acting like a selfish person at

the beginning, because you're not used to putting yourself first. This takes practice, but what I want you to do is spend more time thinking about all the things you love about yourself and less time worrying about other people.

Make a list of things you love about yourself. Come up with as many positive things as you can say about yourself and how amazing you are. Write down all the things you love about your life.

Telling yourself positive things will begin to create a reality in which you constantly feel strong, happy, powerful, confident, active, alive, overjoyed, fulfilled . . .

When your mind is totally focused on how great you feel about yourself, you know what your mind isn't doing? **It's not worrying about what other people think!**

One of the best pieces of advice I have to give is to fill your mind with so many positive things that you're literally too busy to stress over what other people think. Your mind is in a reality where you're already confident and empowered, and there is no need to seek approval from outside yourself. You have created confidence within by actively practicing self-care. Nice job!

Get to a point where what you think about yourself is far more important than what anyone else has to say.

"But if I focus only on myself, won't people think I'm self-centered?"

I thought we weren't worrying about what other people think? Ha ha!

No worries. Self-centered people only think about themselves, right? They tend to be narcissistic and never consider how other people feel. That's not you. If you're reading this book, chances are it's because you're a sensitive, empathic person who cares about people, and that will never go away. Just because you have started practicing self-care doesn't mean you stop caring for others. What it does mean is that you no longer need validation from others to feel good about yourself. You already practice feeling good every day, and you're better at it than anyone.

Now, when you think about other people or help them, you do it because you feel good and helping makes you happy. It's not because you hope they'll return the favor. See how the motivation has changed? This is a good shift and awesome personal growth for the empath or highly sensitive person.

H O M E W O R K

Set the intention to work on yourself this week. For seven days, keep a journal that you update daily. Take notes at work and write down any time you catch yourself worrying about what other people think. Be diligent and keep your notebook handy. You can use your phone to take notes, too, if it's more convenient. Throughout the day, ask yourself questions like, *Do I care what this person thinks? Do I want this person to like me? Am I worrying about what other people think of me?* Be mindful of your thoughts and write them down if your brain is busy trying to please a coworker. After you write down a moment in which you caught your mind wandering, practice letting go.

- Congratulate yourself for paying attention.
- Say affirmations: *I am strong. I am worthy. I deeply love and accept myself. I love feeling joy from within. I am enough.*
- Visualize that good feeling place and describe those emotions again.

- Raise your vibration with activities to look forward to, recite your gratitude list, watch a funny video. Do things that improve your mood.
- Distract your mind with something else.

Do this as often as you can during the day, to train your mind to stay focused on feeling good and confident, while avoiding wondering about other people. At the end of each day, review your notes. What would you improve tomorrow? Where did you knock it out of the park today? Do this every day for a week. Keep writing down instances when you catch yourself dwelling on getting people to like you, and then gently bring your mind back to that good feeling place. At the end of the week, compare your notes. Did you see a decrease in times you thought about the approval of others? Did you get better at calling upon that good feeling place when needed?

The important thing to remember is that this is a lifelong practice. There will be ups. There will be downs. Go easy on yourself and take it one day at a time. The more you train your mind to be independent and self-assured, the less you'll worry about getting people to like you.

"I walked past some coworkers today, and I swear they were talking about me."
Have you ever walked into a room and had the feeling that people were just chatting about you? Have you slightly overheard a conversation at work and thought, *Hey, I think they're talking about me?* This is a common thought, especially for an empath and HSP at work, and how we choose to handle it will affect our mood all day.

There we go again, worrying what other people think. Now our mind is worried that our coworkers were talking smack. Your ego will even grasp at straws trying to convince you this is the truth. *Why did they get quiet as I walked near? They must have been talking about me!* And the ego stirs the pot thicker. This specific paranoid feeling of thinking someone was talking about you stems from the need to be liked—from seeking approval from others. Catch yourself fixating on these thoughts of paranoia and let them go. Don't let your ego be the boss.

Be mindful of your thoughts and pay attention to what your mind is doing. It is not healthy to dwell on negative, hypothetical situations. Be honest with yourself. Do you actually know what was being said, or did you walk past the conversation halfway through and take a few words out of context? Even if a coworker was talking about you, do you have enough information to know whether they were being friendly or hurtful? In any case, it's impossible to know the full conversation without having been there for the whole thing, so let it go.

Our mind is a tool that we can train if we choose. Choose positive, *good feeling* thoughts over hyperanalyzing what you don't know.

If you have ever been in this situation, when you're at work and you could swear someone was just talking about you, shrug your shoulders and drop it. It's not worth worrying about. Oh, and also, why do we tend to think the worst? Is it not more fun to imagine that they were saying supernice things about you? That's way better! It's funny how, through the power of intention, we choose to create scenarios in our minds that can feel good or bad. Choose good scenarios.

20

Raise Your Hand If I Like You

"Life is 10 percent what happens to you and 90 percent how you react to it."
Charles R. Swindoll

In this world, there is never a shortage of jerks ready to ruin your day. But again, keep in mind that each of us has a choice to make when we decide how to handle these people. We decide what to think about. Train your mind to focus on positive, *good feeling* things. Don't dwell on the few bad apples in your orchard of abundance. Fill your basket with the . . . good apples? Weird metaphor, but OK. **Focus on the coworkers you *do* like, not the ones you don't.**

Work is filled with all types. Hard-working types. Quiet types. Stinky types. Mean types. Sensitive types. Always-late types. Sarcasm-as-a-coping-strategy types.

And sensitive people can feel it all. It is incredibly distract-ing having all these people about, talking on their phones, walking behind you, eating their ramen noodles. We have to concentrate if we're going to get any work done at all. A negative emotion is distracting for an empath because we internalize it and process it in the body, like a computer running a self-diagnostic. And if this negative emotion comes from a coworker, it can threaten to consume our thoughts and feelings until we're no longer able to think about anything else. You know that buffering wheel on a computer screen, stuck "thinking" for hours? It's like that, but in the mind. The mind becomes filled with negative thinking and worry and pain. Eventually we associate the whole workplace with this coworker and their negative stuff.

If there are people at work who bug you and make you feel like the entire day is consumed by their energy and your work space feels unbearable—like there is a black cloud hovering as soon as you walk in the door—I get it. You're not alone.

But you can fix this. You can improve your mood and clear the black cloud without changing your reality. You don't need to change their behavior to feel good. Change your perception first.

Why not pay attention to the people you do like at work?

Focus on that good conversation you had with a coworker or that nice thing someone said about your hair. Be mindful and actively look for reasons the people at work are nice. Make a list of the people you do like and keep a mental head count of all the awesome, *good feeling* things that happen at work. This will help train your focus to stay in that good feeling place—giving your attention only to the people who support and honor your well-being. After a time, the bad apples will still be there, but they'll be background noise. Their negative energy will no longer have a grip on you. The buffering wheel will finally be a bar that says "downloading"! Wait, what? Another weird metaphor. But you get it, right?

Stop for a moment and consider what you're thinking about. That terrible coworker? How much they hurt you? How annoying they can be? Tighten your grip on your mind's leash and gently bring it back to how you'd prefer to feel. Let go of thinking about the negative aspects of work and look for reasons to love where you are. Love the cool people you work with. Invite them out for beer and Frisbee golf!

Summary: Watch your thoughts, stop thinking about negative coworkers, and let it go. Focus on the people at work you do like. Consider what you like about them. Come up with reasons you do like work. Write them down and be thankful for everything you can think of. Maybe reach out and build a friendship with someone at work. Establish positive connections with some "good apples" and help reaffirm that work . . . isn't all that bad.

21

How to Take Criticism like a Boss

The empath has a hard time accepting criticism. Most people hear criticism, acknowledge it, and let it fwip by like a stone skipped across the surface of a pond. But empaths absorb all the data around them and process it deeply. The stone sinks to the bottom of the pond to join other random thoughts like *Why does my stomach hurt today?* or *When is the next* Avatar *movie coming out? I wanna live in a tree, too!* We take criticism to heart and analyze it from every angle—like puzzling over that Rubik's Cube we got for Christmas but still can't seem to figure out.

Often the emotions we go through when receiving criticism are dredged up from past experiences. When we hear criticism, it can open the floodgates to old hurt we are still processing, so that one comment at work can feel like a whole lot more. It leaves us feeling drained, depressed, and upset—enveloping our senses in a veritable color palette of emotions. The empath and highly sensitive person has it rough when it comes to criticism.

We can, however, learn to acknowledge and accept criticism in healthy ways. By listening objectively and staying mindful, we're able to avoid latching on to every comment we hear.

"How can I stop taking things personally?"

While I was waiting tables at a restaurant one day, the bartender pulled me aside to tell me that I was ringing in drinks wrong. When I ordered drinks, it had to be no more than four at a time, otherwise he would get overwhelmed. Then he proceeded to say, "You've been here for how long and you don't know this?" He rolled his eyes and slumped off shaking his head, mumbling his disappointment under his breath—as one does when Netflix again raises its monthly fee. I spent the whole day hurting because I honestly didn't know this drink order policy and feared ringing them in again. *That was so mean. Why doesn't he like me?* I mulled.

As a sensitive person, I have the innate ability to overthink things and analyze them to death. It's a gift, really. Not everyone can feel the intolerable injustice done when a coworker simply shrugs at you in the parking lot for no reason. *Were they being friendly, or subversive? I don't get it! What did they mean?* I will overthink these small things and take it so personally that it dominates my mind and ruins my good mood.

But why do we do this? Why does any highly sensitive person or empath take things personally? The signature trait of an empath/ HSP is that they're sensitive to the energy around them. As a generalization, this makes them people pleasers who work very hard to keep those around them happy, safe, and secure. This leads to seeking approval and support from others, from sources outside themselves. When you're dependent on others for your own security, you're setting yourself up for failure, because not everyone has your best interests in mind.

When a coworker acts upset or angry or is mean to them in a direct way, empaths/ HSPs immediately wonder, *What did I do wrong?* They take it personally.

This chapter aims to help you take your power back and recognize that your happiness in life is in your control, not in the hands of anyone else.

Once you become mindful of your thoughts and make the decision to feel happy, you'll realize you can create how you want to feel from within, then project that out into the world and have it reflected back to you. The love and compassion within you is infinite and doesn't rely on any prompting other than your own will to focus on it. After you become mindful, you can detach from the negative, hurtful things your coworkers say and rise above them. You can let them go and learn not to take things personally.

Nothing is more important than how I feel about myself.

All the worry and struggle I've been through to try to fix "what I did wrong" or "what I said" to make this person act like a malicious badger has caused me nothing but pain. In the end, once I practiced building my confidence and joy from within and living in that good feeling place, I found that none of the mean comments at work really mattered. The priority in my life became taking care of myself and focusing on the love I have in my heart—not seeking approval from my coworkers.

My point is, if you're a sensitive person who takes things personally, learn to recognize this part of yourself, get mindful, and let it go. It does no good to wonder why some people say mean things to the point where you get upset and dwell on it. They're not worth your time. It's good to show compassion toward others, but not at the expense of your own well-being. If you start to spiral in negative thoughts, try to catch your thinking mind and stop. Take a deep breath and release it. Think about something else or distract your mind with something so you're not dwelling on those hurtful comments at work. Then, come back to being mindful and feeling elevated when you're ready.

HOMEWORK

- The next time you're at work, pay attention to your trigger points. Who is it? What do they do or say that bothers you so much? Why are you upset? In what way are you taking this personally? Write it down in a notebook.

- Be mindful of your thoughts and catch yourself dwelling on the why, what, when, and how of your coworker's behavior. Breathe. Relax.

- In your mind, say to that person, *You are not in control of my happiness—I am. I accept your comments and criticism and will use them to grow and become a stronger me. I create joy from within.*

- Remember that spending time on hurt and painful thoughts only creates more emotions from the same place. Drop it and let it go. It's time to choose better-feeling thoughts.

- Let things go by breathing, listening to music, calling a friend, getting busy on a project—anything you can do to keep your mind occupied and not overthinking negative situations at work. Reread Chapter 7 for more ideas on how to let things go.

Working with that bartender was tough. Eventually, though, I realized that if it wasn't drinks, it was checks. If it wasn't checks, it was refills or asking "dumb" questions. Nothing I did or said made him happy. This guy was always upset with me and treated me poorly. Over time, I built up confidence by telling myself, *I'm amazing at what I do. I'm happy and personable, and I get compliments and good tips every day. I love myself! I'm done seeking approval from someone who doesn't respect me.* I began looking at this coworker in a new way and decided he'd never be happy. What stuck with me was this: *Nothing I do makes him angry. He's already an angry person. I can't change that, and that's OK.* I started having much better days after that, because his criticism didn't affect me.

"A coworker once told me, 'You need to grow a thick skin and stop being so sensitive.' "

Have you heard this one before? You take time to speak up and communicate how you feel, and your coworker just shrugs it off like it's nothing—like you're the one with the problem. They tell you that you're just too sensitive. "Toughen up! Grow a thick skin!"

Being told that you have to grow a thick skin refers to being able to take criticism and not take things personally.

Having a thick skin means you don't get upset easily, and seemingly nothing bothers you. This is easy for people who don't absorb energy. But sensitive people can't help but internalize and mull deeply over the stimuli in the surrounding environment. It is difficult for the empath/ HSP to just let things go, because we analyze everything and process every detail.

I have never liked this, being told to grow a thick skin. It feels like people who say this are evading taking responsibility for having hurt someone. These people are insecure and don't want to admit they're wrong, and instead tell you, "*You're* the problem. *You* need to change, not me."

This phrase *thick skin* and the implied pointed finger in my face feel like an attack. Since sensitive people tend to take things personally, we do start to question, *Are they right? Am I just not strong enough? Am I too weak for this world?*

Having these thoughts roll around in your head is detrimental to your self-worth. Once you start to question yourself, your mind comes up with ways to reinforce what you're hearing at work. It's not long before other thoughts start knocking at the door, like *I guess I am weak. I am not good enough. I suck.* Now your mind is living completely in such a negative space that it's hard to see any form of confidence left inside. This is the territory of depression and suffering. All because someone at work told you to grow a thick skin.

Be mindful of your thoughts.
You're the only one listening.

Let that negative thinking go. Remind yourself . . .

- You don't need to grow a thick skin. Embrace being sensitive and get back to that good feeling place.
- Take your power back by telling yourself positive things. Use affirmations like I am worthy. *I am strong. I am good enough. I have a right to my opinions. I love myself.*
- Refer to Chapter 9 and remember how great it is to be sensitive. It's a gift.
- If someone tells you to grow a thick skin, say something like, "And lose the part of me that makes me special? No chance!"

Work on improving your confidence and self-worth. Become comfortable being sensitive and treat it like a gift, one that makes you unique and special. Once you do, the commentary in your mind will change, too. *You know . . . I am strong! I feel good enough! I saw Ellen Page at the airport, and she almost looked at me! Life is amazing!* Maybe one day when a coworker tells you to grow a thick skin and laughs, you'll laugh back, thinking how much more aware, spiritually grown, and connected to Spirit you are. That's a comforting thought.

Learning to take criticism is a process. Let's discuss a few scenarios, shall we?

You're Right, I'm Right

So you're driving a bus for the city transit department, and it's up to you to plot the route for the day to be as efficient and effective as possible. A coworker later criticizes your route and suggests what he thinks are better directions. You two argue for while about traffic, rush hour, and school zones before the coworker storms off, telling you how "irkful" you're being. You want to shout back, "First of all, irkful *is not a word. I looked it up. And second, your way isn't better; it's just different!"*

Has this ever happened to you? You do your job correctly, and a coworker tries to pull it apart. Having someone at work go out of their way to judge how you do things and offer unsolicited suggestions is maddening, especially when their aim isn't to educate and help you; it's to feed their own self-driven ego—to boost their self-worth by tearing yours down. These people have a hard time feeling good about themselves on their own, so they drum up outside assistance by hurting and criticizing others.

As a sensitive individual, however, you are more perceptive than most. You can pick up on what people are saying with their words, and the emotions behind them. Observe how your coworker is speaking or trying to criticize or correct you. Does it feel like good advice or merely an attempt to put you down? Allow yourself to smile because you refuse to sway in your confident stature and agree with them just to please their insecure ego. They are not going to win this battle. *Muuaahahaha!*

The insecure coworker will try to sell you that their way is the *right* way of doing things. They'll insist that it's *better* and try to discredit your work any way they can. But you're smart and capable and good-looking. You know perfectly well what you're doing and recognize that their suggestion may be just a *different* way of getting things done, not a better way. Acknowledge their assistance and consider their advice, but be confident in your abilities.

Make changes only if you think your coworker has a valid point. Hold your ground in your opinions and apologize to no one. Ultimately, it's the supervisor, not your idiot coworkers, who will go over your work.

Make alterations at work based on improving yourself, not to placate a coworker's differing opinion.

Listen to your intuition and recognize that a comment or criticism may be either an effort to improve the quality of your work, or an attempt to discredit your methods.

The Coffee Dichotomy

You're at work, where one of your daily tasks is to start the coffeemaker in the morning. Fairly simple; you got this. First the pot gets rinsed out, then a fresh filter and two scoops of coffee get put into the machine before you turn it on. Now, if a customer needs coffee, it'll be ready. Then one day a coworker scolds you for starting the coffee early, saying, "You know you're not supposed to start the coffee until someone asks for it, right?" They huff and grunt with a look of disdain you thought was reserved only for criminals.

So, the next day you skip the coffee and go straight to your next task. The supervisor arrives, notices the coffee machine is sitting untouched, and says, "Why didn't you start the coffee yet? You know that's the first thing you do, right?" They shake their head in disapproval and walk away, leaving you thinking, I can never win. No matter what I do, I get it wrong.

I have countless stories about one person at work telling me to do something, then another coworker coming along and telling me to do the opposite. Then I get chastised by both parties for not following instructions. This always made me feel like a child caught between two parents fighting over how to do my job.

Now, this criticism may stem simply from a coworker who is trying to help you out. To their knowledge, you're not supposed to start the coffee early. That's an honest mistake. But maybe they really are after a way to belittle your efforts to boost their ego. Whatever the reason, this all could have been avoided by simply affirming your confidence in what you are doing.

Say, "Thank you, but I was instructed to do the job this way, and I'm confident I'm doing it right." Done and done. Your coworker may not like this—their bruised ego may take offense. But you've moved past it. Keep focused on how good it feels to be smart, fulfilled, and strong at work. Recite affirmations like *I'm great at what I do. I am worthy. I love and approve of myself deeply. Thank you for this chance to affirm my strength.*

Avoid being a people pleaser and agreeing with whatever criticism comes your way. Think about your coworker's comment and decide whether it warrants any action. If you have questions about a particular task, go to the source and ask your supervisor for more clarification. But if you feel self-assured in your poise on the job, stand firm and let your coworker know. When you do, remember, this moment isn't for you to dwell on how your coworker's feelings must be hurt. Focus again on that good feeling place, reaffirm your self-confidence, and let your inner voice sing. Pat yourself on the back for being assertive and not giving them the attention they're looking for.

Now, you can start the coffee whenever you darn well please.

Doing 100 Things Right

It's a 12-hour shift in the mechanic's bay. You're surrounded by noisy engines and puddles of oil, dirt, and grime, and the smell of gasoline hangs in the air, threatening to veil the other stink of exhaust fumes. Today you have to sweep the floors; organize machine parts on shelves; clean pistons; install new spark plugs, wires, and a distributor cap (but first you must learn what a distributor cap is); and wash and rinse seven trucks.

You get all this done in record time and feel such a sense of accomplishment you want to glide across the floor like Tom Cruise in Risky Business, *but with pants. As you're completing a final task, a coworker approaches and claims that you forgot to put some parts away. Their tone is filled with frustration and anger. And you think,* You don't want to say thank you for all the hundred other things I did today? No, you want to point out the one thing I missed? Cool.

Sometimes our coworkers can be in a bad mood and express that stress outwardly. Maybe that criticism about putting parts away was really stress about something else, in which case, let it go. Use your gift of perception and see if they've just been in a sour mood all day and the parts thing was just another chip in the mirror. Or do you have someone at work who only speaks to you to point out your mistakes? It's as if these people lie in wait, looking for an opportunity to correct you—like a panther ready to lunge.

Because you're a sensitive person who feels more

deeply than others, this criticism can blindside you. You might think, *No one says thank you to me for taking out the trash, or compliments my great presentation I worked so hard on. But I miss one thing and all of a sudden they have something to say. What the heck?*

It's like you can do 100 things right at work, but that one thing you miss is a world crisis. Some coworkers love to point out flaws in others. Why is this? One reason, again, is the ego. The ego is looking for ways to feel superior. Jumping at a chance to criticize someone at work is a weak-minded attempt to boost how they feel by tearing you down. Notice how these certain people tend to never speak up to compliment you on a good job. It's because a narcissist thinks only of themselves. They're not about to lift anyone up with praise because that would elevate those around them. And the ego-mind can't have that. Pay attention to the narcissists at your workplace and avoid them as best you can.

Oh, narcissists, you poor souls. Find someone else to feed off of, will you?

If you find someone at work who seems to criticize you for any reason, there are ways to approach the emotions you feel in a healthy, constructive manner. Follow some of these suggestions.

- Slap them in the face and walk away slowly to "Uptown Funk" by Bruno Mars. (*Totally kidding!*)

Some constructive ways to manage criticism:

1. Breathe deeply a few times and become calm. Taking criticism is hard for sensitive people. You're not alone.
2. Be mindful of your thoughts and don't cling to the coworker's criticism. Reread Chapter 7 to practice letting go. Get to that good feeling place as often as you can.
3. Listen carefully to what your coworker is saying and acknowledge them. It's always good to practice being polite.
4. Decide whether or not to act on their advice. Should you feel confident you're doing the job correctly, say thank you and let them know you'll take it under advisement. If need be, assert your voice and tell them flat out, "I feel like my way works just fine. If I have questions, I'll let you know."
5. Holding your ground and being assertive can be hard for sensitive people. We need practice. Reread Chapter 15 for assistance.
6. Some affirmations are . . .

- I am great at my job.
- I am fantastic at what I do.
- I am worthy.
- I got a compliment the other day that felt really good.
- I am confident in my abilities.
- I create how I want to feel, and I feel amazing.

7. Remind yourself that this coworker feeds off of your emotional turmoil. They are weak and self-conscious, because they need you to make them feel good about themselves. Take comfort in the fact that as a sensitive person, you're stronger than that. You're a rock star with emotions! Use your gift to create and build the reality you choose to feel from within.

8. Do your happy dance.

Once you become comfortable standing up for yourself and you don't budge when your coworker tries to criticize you, they'll start to back off. They will learn you're no longer the easy target they thought you were. Now they have to look somewhere else to feed their ego.

22

A Mountain or a Molehill

Scenario: Claire is an empath working as a ticket agent at a train station. She's good at her job, is never late, and is kind and courteous with guests. One day a passenger arrives at the ticket desk huffing under his breath, with narrowed eyes like a hawk's and a scowl you'd expect at 3 a.m. on a rainy train platform. His bad mood stretches ahead like a dark-clouded envoy, reaching Claire before they exchange pleasantries. The passenger begins by quietly explaining all the travel mishaps, delayed flights, lost reservations, and traffic that have led him to seek a train at 3 in the morning. He demands, planting his thick forefinger into the ticket window, to be taken care of immediately—all while never raising his voice above a church whisper.

Although Claire is busy attending to the guest's inquiries, her mind is reeling with panic, and her chest tightens as she copes with this sudden influx of emotion. Later on . . .

"How was the morning, Claire?" a coworker asks.

"It was awful! This guy totally screamed at me this morning and demanded a million things!"

I don't know how many people out there do this as well, but I'm guilty of exaggerating a story at work, saying that I was "yelled at" by my boss, when in truth it may have been more like forceful, direct communication—not "yelling," per se. Have you ever felt like someone at work yelled at you? Did they really yell, or do you just feel that way? It's important to know which.

It's interesting how sensitive people perceive the world. What we hear and see and what we perceive can often be two different things. We don't just take things at face value, we feel the underlying emotion attached to people, places, media, and so on. This is a gift, like being able to use x-ray vision to see what's really going on. But being sensitive people also means we are deep thinkers, and we internalize events and replay them in our minds. The longer we analyze an event or, rather, feel an emotion, the more power it gains—like a snowball barreling down a hill, getting bigger and bigger. It is common to grow over-whelmed by these thoughts and emotions, and if we're not careful, our minds will run away with these emotions and turn what started as a molehill into a mountain.

In the workplace, many of us are part of a team. That means we all have to work together and help one another. Some people are better teachers than others. They can approach you with compassion and understanding and explain things in a simple, easy-to-understand manner. These people make work a nice place to be. Think Mr. Rogers doing a safety briefing in the conference room. Yellow sweater and all!

Still, there are those individuals who seem to have no people skills. They can be abrasive, loud, irritating, and even insulting. Working with these people is not easy for a sensitive empath, because we absorb all their pain and negativity. It can *feel* like an exercise in daily torture. It can feel like they're yelling at us. Although they may be speaking in a calm, collected voice, because their message carries an emotional trigger of some kind, it feels like their energy is shouting. It's overwhelming and draining for empaths and highly sensitive people.

Being the deep thinkers that we are, our minds love to take this negativity and replay it over and over again, letting it snowball as we even create hypothetical situations to reinforce this shouting we feel. This is the ego taking control. The ego feels hurt and wants attention, so it creates a reality in which it plays the victim. This is dangerous ground, because the mind may begin to distort reality until we really only see what we want to see. When it comes time to describe the event or person at work that upset us, we may be so worked up for so long that it can be difficult to pinpoint the truth.

Slow down and back that train up.

When a coworker upsets you, it's important to separate fact from fiction. Be honest with yourself and state facts. Were they actually yelling? What words did they actually use? When you replay this event in your head or to others, are you exaggerating for effect? Is your ego taking control and begging for attention?

Shouldering responsibility for how you feel takes a lot of courage. No one wants to point the finger at themselves and say, "I'm the problem. I need to change." It's much easier to blame the colleague at work when you feel cruddy, but your attitude and perception every day are choices you make. How you feel depends on you, not your environment.

I think empaths/ HSPs have a tendency to use harsh, exaggerated vocabulary to describe hurtful people because we want to get the point across that we were deeply hurt. We want to use words that better express how we feel.

So we use *yell* instead of *talk* because that's the emotion we associate with what upset us. And we're afraid if we don't exaggerate, no one will pay attention. It can become a habit to embellish events to the point where you don't even realize you're doing it.

Again, this is all the ego-mind vying for attention and trying to feed a bottomless pit of insecurity. It wants to play the victim to receive pity, support, sympathy, love . . . We all have an ego, but learning to quell its childish temper tantrums is the first step toward accepting *what is*, allowing the present moment to just be so you can invite that good feeling place to fill your entire being.

One of the many burdens we must bear as sensitive people is that not everyone will understand how we feel. We can try to explain it, but most people don't share the same level of empathy, so it feels like talking to an open refrigerator. No feedback, cold, smells like salad dressing . . .

Let go of trying so hard to convince others of how you feel. Your feelings are already valid, because you are you. You exist, you're here in this world, and you have as much right to your emotions as the next person. There is no need to exaggerate events in the hope that others will feel your emotions, too. Work on being more confident and secure within yourself. Become a person who needs no outside validation: you create strength and self-worth from within.

Learn to distinguish between facts and what your mind wants to perceive.

Don't create a mountain out of a molehill.

23

Workplace Drama

Take notice of which people drain you, and avoid them as much as you can.

Some coworkers love drama, don't they? Spouting gossip about Jan or spreading rumors about Mike, just to feel a false sense of superiority. They feed off it like a fruit bat in a mango tree. They are begging for your attention, and they come to you because you're the best listener. You'll give them the most attention. (Attention feels like support, and support feels like love. These coworkers have found an unhealthy, hurtful way to feel love.) But while they feed their egos and talk drama, you become drained and exhausted. Yuck.

Run from these people like a flash flood warning!

I see two things happening here:

EMPATH AT THE OFFICE

1. **It's distracting.** Listening to a coworker talk nonstop about irrelevant drama is one of the ultimate distractions at work. You know those feelings of anxiousness, tension, stress, or maybe worry and panic you may be struggling with? Those feelings increase and run amok in our brains when we're distracted. To avoid those emotions, we have to practice a high degree of self-awareness. Unhealthy, long-term distractions that keep our minds from paying attention to the self knock us off center. Listening to a coworker's drama and incessant talking is one of the big ones to get away from as much as you can.

    Sensitive people, more than others, need to be mindful of this drama, so they don't get distracted and slip into a disconnected state—one in which a person's mind is so distracted by stimuli that they are no longer aware of or working with their body. They become ungrounded and detached from that "centered" feeling of awareness. Most people live like this, but you're reading this book and trying to balance yourself. Good on you!

2. **It's negative.** The second thing I see is the energy of this drama at work. Have you noticed how you feel

when these people talk trash about everyone else? It feels gross and ugly. It's such negative energy to listen to someone say ugly things about the people you work with. Empaths feel this negative energy more profoundly. We absorb this negative drama unwittingly into our bodies and then walk around with it all day, trying to process this extra weight. It's horrible.

If your coworker is laying on a thick layer of negative drama:

- **Practice mindfulness.** Your coworker is competing for your attention. They want you to be distracted so you'll focus only on them. Don't fall for it. Don't let them distract you from paying attention to the self and staying that calm, cool version of yourself you love so much.

- **Avoid them.** Plain and simple. If you don't have to be around them, go find a safe place away from their exhausting energy.

- **Set boundaries.** Know what you're comfortable with, and if someone at work pushes past your boundaries, tell them. Say, "Excuse me, that's not a very nice thing to say." Or maybe, "I don't mean to interrupt, but could we change the subject?" Or you can suggest something more casual to talk about, like, "If you could have any superpower, what would it be?"

There will always be drama, no matter where you work. And there will be people who feed off drama and want to blabber about it to you. Don't get caught up in the drama at work.

24

If You Can't Beat 'Em . . .

Have you ever worked with someone who teased you constantly? It's not that they were being mean per se, but this was how they showed affection. As if making fun of you meant they liked you? What a stupid way to be! If you like someone, just be nice! Anyway . . .

There is plenty of good-natured banter at work that is meant to be completely harmless. Some people poke fun or tease as if to illustrate the sense of camaraderie they feel toward you. As if to say, "I'm comfortable around you. Let's be friends." Even so, sometimes an empath/ HSP can have a difficult time accepting this light teasing and letting it go. It hurts. And what's more, these coworkers seem oblivious to whether they upset someone.

First of all, learn to be more assertive and not to take things so personally. These skills will benefit you at work and in your personal life as well. Once you begin to feel more assertive, put it into practice by giving as good as you get.

If you can't beat 'em, join 'em.

All the good-natured ribbing being tossed back and forth between coworkers is typically not an HSP's preferred style of affection, but you can decide, *Hey, if this is the environment I find myself in, I might as well tease and poke fun back.* Doing so can make you feel like part of the group and help you fit in and be in the family. You can tell yourself, *I'll accept this behavior for now, and if they cross a line, I'll let them know. But until then, if they talk sh--, I will, too!* This practice showcases your confidence and security in yourself. Keep it light and friendly. No need to go overboard.

Some people know how to tease affectionately, with completely harmless intentions—like you do with your family. But other people can be too crass and even downright offensive. This is where you could draw the line and either speak up and tell them to knock it off, or confide in a friend for comfort. If you do feel the need to speak up and assert yourself, do it sooner rather than later. If you let them tease you for weeks or months on end, they learn that this behavior is OK. It becomes harder for them to change. But the first time they cross a line and you let them know, they'll be more inclined to stop.

Also, if someone at work really isn't getting the hint that their teasing bothers you, just avoid them. They aren't worth being around if they make you feel bad, so just walk the other way.

Why do some people choose to tease and make fun of others? There are so many reasons why someone would act this way and be motivated to poke fun at people. Maybe they just want you to feel like part of the family. Perhaps it's a defense mechanism they've developed. If they're busy cracking jokes and teasing those around them, no one can see just how vulnerable they really feel. Their humor keeps people at a distance.

Use your best judgment when lightheartedly teasing a coworker or friend. Have fun with it and enjoy the emotion of camaraderie.

Conclusion

That's it. That's all I've got. This little book is the culmi-
nation of everything I have learned and put into practice in
my life to improve my confidence and happiness at work.
All these techniques and tools, I worked on through trial
and error until I found I was living the version of myself
I wanted to be. One day I just looked at my life and said,
"Hey, look at how much happier I am. I guess this stuff
works!" Not only did my attitude at work change for the
better, but I improved my relationships with my family,
my friends, and even strangers I meet. I can stand in line
at a crowded bank, and where I used to feel panicked and
claustrophobic from all the bodies standing too close, now
I feel joyful and content just to let them be. It's a choice
I make to guide my thoughts toward happiness and fun. I
love the new me.

It is my sincerest hope that this book has helped you
in some way. I feel there are many gems in here that can
teach empaths and highly sensitive people to become

better versions of themselves: to become strong, powerful warriors of emotion and navigate this life like you're standing at the bow of some great ship, feeling the ocean air with your arms spread wide, inviting new challenges and opportunities from up ahead. You're wearing slacks from the early 1900s, and maybe you won your ticket in a poker game . . . No, wait—that's *Titanic*.

Suggested Reading

- *Breaking the Habit of Being Yourself: How to Lose Your Mind and Create a New One*, by Dr. Joe Dispenza
- *The Empath's Survival Guide: Life Strategies for Sensitive People*, by Judith Orloff, MD
- *Feeling Is the Secret*, by Neville Goddard
- *A Gradual Awakening*, by Stephen Levine
- *Infinite Self: 33 Steps to Reclaiming Your Inner Power*, by Stuart Wilde
- *Intuition Medicine: The Science of Energy*, by Francesca McCartney
- *The Intuitive Way: The Definitive Guide to Increasing Your Awareness*, by Penny Peirce
- *The Power of Now: A Guide to Spiritual Enlightenment*, by Eckhart Tolle
- *You Can Heal Your Life*, by Louise Hay

WEBSITES

www.opencurrentlife.com
www.ambleunbound.com

Made in the USA
Coppell, TX
26 June 2021